AF409682

With Tales and Folly Instead of Pills

by Andrew Levitt

Dedication

With gratitude to all the patients and families I have seen and to all the doctors, nurses, staff and volunteers with whom I have worked,

with special thanks to Susan, my guardian angel in Pediatrics, who has had the wisdom not to protect me from making a complete fool of myself.

In deference to her influence and importance to me and my work, I mention my childhood pediatrician by name in Chapter One. Everywhere else, in order to protect the privacy of individuals, no actual names or identifying details are used in this book.

Contents

With Tales and Folly Instead of Pills

Dr. Merryandrew: All my stories are old stories, not because they were told long ago or because they are about things that happened long ago. They are old stories because I learned from the old masters. The old masters knew that life was full of magic and miracle. They knew that animals could turn into people and people could turn into animals; that any path goes down before it goes up and it goes through darkness before it comes to light. They knew we meet many guides and helpers in our lives. Some of these are guides we seek. Some are helpers who show up when we think we are lost, stuck and alone. Sometimes they help us by doing what we ask. Sometimes they guide us by asking us to do something for them. Maybe if we listen to the old stories, we will know what the old masters knew. Maybe if more people hear the old stories, there will be more people around who know that life is full of magic and miracle.

Dr. Merryandrew

I don't know if there are those who bring appreciation for magical consciousness, the sincerity in wit, and the wisdom born of dreaming to a story about a clown who spends part of every day in a hospital dressed in a lab coat, pork pie hat, bowtie, and clown nose. I do know a number of people feel a clown must be hiding something behind the mask of a painted smile or red nose. They ascribe to all clowns malevolent character concealed beneath the cheerful facade. They expect no better from a clown in the hospital. Some whom I have met as patients or parents of patients bristle when I stick my head into a hospital room. They will not have me come in. Though it is not a common experience, I have had the rare nurse turn her back on me in the staff elevator and measure her breathing until the elevator arrived at the floor where she could escape the imputed danger. Some doctors with a sense of the high seriousness of their profession, I suppose, ignore my cheerful greeting in the hall as if they disdain association with the likes of me.

Generally, however, I am well received with a welcoming smile. I find most doctors and nurses to be supporters and better than that, true colleagues. Indeed, wittingly or unwittingly, the doctors and nurses with whom I work often become participants in my folly. And certainly I have found patients and families aplenty who welcome me into hospital rooms and join in my improvisations. I will have something to say later on to those patients, nurses and doctors who express their disapproval, but only by way of acknowledgment. I have no animus in that regard. In fact, I am grateful that they have kept me alert to how I am received. They remind me that my place in healthcare is not a given. It must be circumscribed by care and listening to the patients and families and other fellow human beings whom I encounter as I make my rounds in the hospital.

I will have a bit more to say to those who have had enough interest to ask me how I got into this business of being a medical clown and those who have said "It must be moving to do what you do" or simply, "Thank you for what you do." I feel in the acknowledgment a nod of approval.

I appreciate it. Nevertheless, while I will offer in some pages that follow an explanation of how I came to this work and where I stand in it, I do not intend this book to be a personal defense or a book about me. I have a simple mantra that I recite to myself in the hospital repeatedly, "It is not about me. Listen!" Accordingly, this is a book about what I have found to offer as I have sensed and heard from patients what gives them a feeling of lightness and well-being. As such, this book is written for those who might ask with a bit of an edge, "What is this clown doing in the hospital?" and for those who say in one way or another, "It is good to see a clown in the hospital. Tell me about what you do."

Little did I know when I began on April Fool's Day many years ago in this middle-sized city hospital in North Carolina that I would journey through the antiseptic halls and rooms of a hospital into the verdant landscape around the soul and the dark and clear recesses to be found within it. Little did I expect that in hospital rooms with IV poles ticking and monitors clocking vital signs that I would discover moments that inspire reverence and awe for the mystery that abounds in all beings and things. I began like anyone with the understanding that health is defined by physiological function and is measured by blood tests and vital signs. I humbly thought an emotionally positive presence might serve to sweeten the medicine or distract from discomfort. Of course, I did allow that perhaps in time I would discover that there was more to it than that.

After seeing patients day-to-day for many years now, I have come to understand that there is another definition of health. In this other definition, health does not just refer to the status of the physical body. This other definition of health incorporates the status of the soul and the soul's capacity to engage another and the mystery inherent in living. Health may be measured with laughter, as well as with seriousness. It may be met with a light heart, as well as solemnity. It is a quality that cannot be quantified, but we can know it and sense it in ourselves and recognize it in others as a positive state of well-being. Absence of pain or infection is not the only measure of health; health may also be encountered and expressed as a sense of beauty, a sense of humor, appreciation of music and song, as alignment with the animal and vegetable kingdoms of nature, as the capacity to imagine, as the ability and willingness to be drawn into the tensions of a story, and, of course, as acknowledgement and response to another.

Although in our compartmentalized age, religion, psychology, anthropology, and aesthetic theory might lay different claims in this territory of which I write, I believe all would be well served to maintain a lack of departmental distinctions and consider well-being as a comprehensive whole.

One day a patient complaining of abdominal pain arrived in the Pediatric Emergency Department. I was able to see her before the doctor could get to her room. During the twenty minutes or so we spent together, I found her very receptive. She cheerfully participated in an exchange with my alter ego, who inhabits a marionette clown. He sang and danced; she laughed. They bantered about a Wonderland where all ones wishes come true. She volunteered a wish or two she would like to see fulfilled. Later in the morning, I noticed that the doctor had ordered the standard appendicitis work-up. I caught the doctor passing the nurses' station and asked, "Do you really think she's an appy (an emergency room abbreviation for an appendicitis patient)?" The doctor responded, "In my heart of hearts, No." I agreed, "I have never seen a patient come in here with appendicitis who could respond as she did." Our hunches were confirmed by blood work and X-rays. Of course, in saying this, I am not claiming to be a diagnostician.

Nor am I suggesting that the doctor should have listened to her heart and not ordered the tests and X-rays. If she had no other reason, the Hippocratic Oath requires that patients be offered the best medical treatment available. At this time in history, the best medical evaluation includes radiographs and quantitative measures. They are standards of common protocol. Nevertheless, I use this instance to illustrate that the doctor and I both, by different means to be sure, recognized immeasurable signs of well-being. If I hadn't asked her, the doctor would likely have discounted her heart altogether. That is a part of her training. In this instance, there could be no significant consequence to ignoring the heart's hunch. I suspect, however, that doctors who have been in their profession a while have seen instances where the medical measures and the mysterious quality of well-being seemed irreconcilable. About those instances, some doctors might admit mystery's indications were borne out. In more instances than we know, a positive or negative sense of well-being may open or close an alternative path of healing. As I said, most doctors and caretakers of patients and all of us who have observed life well know health is not solely a quantifiable measure of function. Somewhere in our lives as patients or caring for another who is ill, we have discovered the truth that there is a distinction between not being sick and a positive sense of well-being, and the distinction is not merely one of degree, but may be more on the order of category and type.

§ § §

Early on, when the assistant director of Pediatrics gave me a tour around the unit, we stopped at the bedside of one patient she had known his whole life. Because I was in my street clothes, she told him who I was. He heard what I was going to be doing and immediately responded, "Great idea. Sort of like a therapy dog." Contrary to expectations otherwise, I did not feel demeaned. In fact, I was deeply honored by the comparison, with reason. When my old dog died, my vet consoled me with a story about a child she knew. This child had also lost a much loved dog, but her parents noticed she was not sad. When they asked her how she felt about her dog, she said she understood why he was gone. Dogs, she said, live shorter lives than people do because the purpose of life is to learn to love. Dogs know that is the purpose of life and they are born knowing how to love.

Sometimes I feel I may be considered a poor substitute for a therapy dog. After all, dogs are recognized as therapy. By contrast, I know there are those who regard me with suspicion or at best, a mixture of mischief, fluff and circus sawdust. I am not unfamiliar with being treated as unreal. When I used to perform as a mime at the yearly furniture market and at street festivals, people would sometimes pinch or punch me to see if I could feel and speak. One man threw darts at me as if I were a moving target at the fair and no one warned him off his game. Nevertheless I have never been dissuaded from sharing what I do with purpose. If a child's perspective can be trusted, which I believe it can, I share a sense of life's purpose with dogs.

§ § §

I am standing outside the door of a room in the Pediatric unit. It is a hot 90° summer day. The thermostat I just passed in the hall said it is 74° inside. Inside the hospital, it is always the same indefinable season. It is easy to forget the weather and the season in here. Everyone is accustomed to leaving the natural world at the door as they enter. It is part of our expectation of hospital medicine that it takes place in a controlled atmosphere. But today, I am noticing the difference between outside and in. Although today in particular, I am noticing the difference at the thermostat, in one way or another I always bring awareness of the outside in with me. It is a habit with me since I have spent a lot of time outdoors in raw landscapes and cultivated spaces, in the remote and near, threatening and soothing, startling and ordinary wildness of life. For at least the last twenty years, as well, I have tried to align myself with the rhythms of the natural world and to cultivate a sensibility for the more-than-human-world: the caterwaul of crows at dawn, the rasp of the heron's call as it oars the air above a creek, the piercing screech of a solitary hawk at the edge of the woods, the sociability of the titmouse and the chickadee in the backyard, the silent concentrated intensity within the fox's eye, the frivolity of daffodils and the grace of dogwoods in the spring, the long-suffering patience of oaks, the doleful brooding of dark cumulous clouds, the rainbow's joyful enthusiasm for refracted light. I have come to feel the terror of the rabbit at the hypnotizing cry of the owl in the dark, the tremble of the dog when the thunder cracks, and the scream of the trees when ice breaks their limbs. I ground myself in the moods of the living earth. So in that sense you could say, I am an outsider inside in the hospital.

On the long walk in from the main entrance to the elevator, I use the time to settle into life in the interior of the hospital. I try to relinquish what has held my attention on the outside and notice the mood of people in the surgical waiting area, which is located along the entrance hall. I greet and smile to those who are waiting there and stop to talk if anyone calls me over. Gradually, I take up the life of a clown who lives in the immediacy of each moment.

This is the very first door that I stood before when I first came to the hospital on April 1st, 2011. It probably seems like a deliberate choice that I started on April Fool's Day, but it was not. It just happened that my background checks, shots and TB test caught up with me in time for me to perform at an outdoor event planned by the Pediatric unit of the hospital to initiate Child Abuse Awareness Month and then to come into the unit afterward on the same day to begin my "clown rounds," room-to-room visits with patients. Now nine years on, I have not forgotten the trepidation with which I stood before this door on that first day. Just before I knocked on the door to gain entry, I froze and asked myself, "What are you going to do when you get into the room?" My answer to myself was, "I don't know. I may have a lot of skills developed over many years of performing, but I don't know how those skills will serve me in the hospital one-on-one with patients." I worried to myself, "What did I get myself into?" But I grasped at a straw of courage and knocked on the door, knowing as I knocked that I was going to have to pretend confidence and competence I did not feel and hope in the pretending that I would find my way with improvisation. Nevertheless in those first moments, it was mostly bluff and blunder.

Maybe not entirely bluff and blunder. At least, I was prepared to introduce myself when I entered the room. I had anticipated that I was going to have to indicate to patients and families immediately upon entry that I was there for their pleasure. I would not be delivering shots or pills; I would not be palpating the patient's abdomen or giving a probing exam. Nor was I there to make anyone feel foolish; as the fool in the room, folly was mine to own. I intended no harm. To make all this clear, I had written a bit of doggerel, which I printed on a badge and could recite as I entered the room.

Dr. Merryandrew

I am the doctor who treats your ills
with tales and folly instead of pills.

On the bottom of the badge, I gave a dictionary style definition of merryandrew:

(mer-ree-an-drew), noun: a clown; a buffoon; a person who amuses others by ridiculous behavior.

Thus I began my first visit to a patient's room with the words I had prepared to recite. I hoped that even if young patients did not understand what the words meant, they would pick up from the lilt and rhyme that I was playful. Since that first visit, I have begun all my visits to patients with those same words. Only once in nine years did a patient's curious response take me aback. After I introduced myself, BJ, a three-year-old girl in an Emergency Department room, asked me, "Do you have a tail?" Nonplused, I responded, "No. Do you?" Then on the back swing, with the help of BJ's mother, I caught with delight the pun my introduction seems to *entail*.

§ § §

If Dr. Merryandrew's words of introduction were but slight glimmer of his emerging persona, they were yet light enough in which to clothe myself and to sense the doctor's manner as I looked in the mirror. Although these days many doctors in the hospital forgo the white coat as the uniform of the profession, I knew I wanted to evoke that old tradition to distinguish my clown as a doctor. I counted on the clown nose, pork pie hat and bow tie over a colorful T-shirt to mitigate the sterile austerity of the white coat by signaling I was an advocate of fun. I chose to wear only the clown nose to minimize the impersonality and distance a make-up mask can convey. If there was some ambiguity in the image I presented, neither recognizable as a medical doctor nor identifiable as a usual clown, it was intentional.

Over the years some people have puzzled over the ambiguity and asked me, "Are you a doctor?" When the question seemed to come from a bemused adult, I have responded, "Yes, I am your doctor. I am the doctor who treats your ills with tales and folly instead of pills." But if the questioner was genuinely inquiring, I have responded, "Yes, but not a medical doctor. I am a Ph.D." But I have tried to avoid saying more about my doctorate in Folklore from Penn because any further information about my academic background would detract from the indefinable potentiality of Dr. Merryandrew's image. I have not wanted to allow him to be labeled and dismissed or to be fixed with a credential.

As a clown, I wanted to signal that Dr. Merryandrew is neither heir to Harlequin with his slapstick and broad pranks nor to Harlequin's shadow partner, Pierrot, the bumbling dreamer. I would wear neither the multicolored face-paint of the august clown of the circus, nor the clown white of the stage and street mime. Although I had worn whiteface for some of my performances in my career, I also used masks I created myself and my red-nosed clown character wore no make-up. My status among clowns was in the broad category of Eccentrics, clowns whose clowning adheres to no type. When I was performing in a theater festival in Atlanta in 1990, I was identified among Eccentrics as a "Cosmic Clown." The category was conceived by Benny Reehl, who was then a well-known director of New Vaudeville in New England, and he placed me in the category as its sole proprietor. Benny called me a "cosmic clown" because my symbolic play grew out of reflections on grand themes concerning the place of humans in the universe and the meaning of life on Earth. Perhaps the titles of my shows will give some indication that they were created to tease the audience toward reflection and depth. My frequently performed show for children was titled, "Stick to Your Dreams, Don't Go in the Lion's Cage and Make a Little Mischief Every Day." My first full-length show was "Mimes of Innocence and Experience," and the last show I created was "Hooligan, or the Fool and his Scepter," a symbolic journey through transformations of unconscious Shadow grotesqueries into the joyful wisdom of a fool. I sensed that my clown doctor was to be a manifestation of my cosmic clown, but I did not know how that would develop in the persona of Dr. Merryandrew as I gave birth to the doctor.

I put a small flashlight in the breast pocket of the lab coat, a stethoscope in the left hip pocket and a kazoo and rhythm egg in the right hip pocket for possible use in improvisation with patients. I clipped the name badge with its introductory couplet to the right lapel of the coat and decided I was suitably attired to present myself in the hospital.

I felt, however, that to complete my image, I needed a bag. I imagined an old style black leather doctor's bag of the kind I remembered my pediatrician brought with her when she made house calls. But alas, doctors who make house calls are uncommon these days and consequently, the doctor bag is mostly considered a thing of the past or so rare an object in use that it is prohibitively expensive to purchase. I considered contemporary variations on the shape of the doctor bag made of canvas or nylon, but they had none of the magic or mystique of the old bags. To be practical and expeditious, I looked around my house and happened on a make-up chest in my closet. My wife had given me the chest when I was performing regularly, but I felt it was too large for the make-up I carried when I was traveling. So the chest was unused.

It is rectangular in shape measuring 10 x 16 inches and 8 ½ inches deep. It is constructed on a board base covered on the outside by what could be woven willow darkly stained. The edges are trimmed with leather; the eight corners are capped with brass; three brass clasps hold the lid closed; and there is a carrying handle in the middle of the top of the case. The inside of the box is covered with fabric that can be wiped. As I said my choice of the chest was practical and expeditious. What I discovered, however, was that the chest had its own mystique. It looked like an object out of another time when it was brand new and with time and many cleanings with hospital wipes, it now has an antique look. When I walk into rooms these days, children often ask, "What's in the treasure box?" By now it has been filled with the magical objects of my trade, but in those initial days, I carried the chest simply as an accessory for Dr. Merryandrew. In lab coat, pork pie hat, bow tie over colorful T-shirt, and clown nose, with the chest clasped in his left hand, the image of Dr. Merryandrew was complete and he was ready to knock on the first door of a patient room in the hospital.

Chapter One

The Magical Doctor's Bag and the Treasure Chest

I am happy that Dr. Merryandrew's "treasure chest" has been incorporated in patients' magical consciousness for the image of an old leather doctor's bag from which it derived has been a magical object in my consciousness since my childhood and I had hoped to evoke the powers of the original. The doctor's bag of my childhood was carried by my own pediatrician when she made house calls.

Dr. Elsa Farmer was a slight German woman with a serious austere look characteristic of many in her nation of origin and in her profession at the time. Her clothes never had any color that I can remember. In my memory, she wore only black skirts and white blouses. Her hair, pulled back in a bun or by barrettes, was gray during all the years she was my doctor. And she peered at me from behind wireless glasses. Nothing in the description would seem to be reassuring to a child. Yet she had an aura of confidence and competence and she exuded the trustworthiness of one dedicated to a life of caring for others. As a child, I sensed all that and felt comfortable with her.

I was too young to ever learn anything about her life then, but I know she was a child of turn of the century Germany and I assume she received her medical training in Germany. That means she would have been trained in the very best scientific medicine of her day. She probably came to the United States sometime before or after World War I, probably after since she was married to an American.

It was a different era in medicine. Medicine, certainly pediatric medicine, was still a cottage industry. Penicillin was a new discovery and all of us in my family were allergic to it. The Salk polio vaccine was not tested on us until my age group was in the second or third grade when we received inoculations *en masse* at school. Many of the medicines we used were the legacy of antiquity – iodine, mercurochrome, ichthamol, aspirin. I remember having my throat swabbed with iodine. Bed rest was the primary prescription for most ills. As patients we acceded to the doctor's unquestioned authority and rested, drank weak tea, and ate toast with grape jelly.

Dr. Farmer's office was in a wood frame house with a small front porch across the street from my elementary school. You walked in the front door and turned to the left to enter the small waiting room to the office. There were toys in a basket to play with, some child-sized chairs and adult-sized chairs for sitting. Hanging on the wall in the center of the waiting room was a framed print of Renoir's painting of a child holding a watering can in what looks like a summer garden. The child wore a dark black dress trimmed with lace. For all the years I sat in that waiting room up through the age of 14, I assumed the child in the painting was Dr. Farmer when she was a young girl.

The overall impression of the office itself was sterile white — white enamel surfaces, white cabinets and closets, white sink and white tiled bathroom, a white table as a desk, and, of course, a white scale of the old style with a yard stick built into it to measure height. For that measurement, I always tried to stretch myself up to my greatest height. On the back wall there was an early primitive X-ray machine that we children only understood to be a crude wooden vise for the human body that sandwiched us between two boards while our picture was taken. In this office I received the immunizations available at the time. Dr. Farmer delivered shots painlessly. Even in the last year that I saw her before she retired because her hands were crippled with rheumatoid arthritis, she could deliver a painless shot by holding the syringe in one curled fist and pushing the plunger with the palm of the other hand. I was also brought to the office occasionally for lacerations that needed the doctor's attention.

On rare occasions that I can no longer account for, I was allowed to enter the room to the right of the front door. To the right was a room from another world, the Old World. The Oriental rug, leather couch and piano seemed antiquated, objects steeped in the mysteries of another era. But what I remember most vividly about that room was that the three walls that did not have windows looking out to the road were lined with books, bookcases from ceiling to floor . Most astonishing to my childhood imagination was that the door through which I entered the room was part of the bookcase. When it was closed the entrance was hidden. That door made the room an enchanted space, a contrast to the sterile atmosphere of the office. I would have liked to visit that room more times than I did. But I went infrequently to the doctor's house. For illness was attended at home.

As a child, whenever I felt fatigued, coughed, had a fever or a rash, my temperature was taken with the mercury thermometer and I was put to bed. Dr. Farmer was called. We never knew how many others she would be visiting during her visiting hours or where we were in the list. During the wait, I felt a degree of anxiety. But when the doorbell rang and a moment later I heard her soft German accent downstairs, I was always relieved. She came up the stairs into the bedroom, threw down her black trench coat on a rainy day or her wool greatcoat in winter at the end of the bed, sat down at my side and put her black leather doctor's bag beside her. Out of the bag came the diagnostic instruments, the stethoscope, pressure cuff, otoscope/ophthalmoscope, reflex hammer. All these seemed like magical instruments to me for they allowed the doctor to look and listen to a life inside of me about which I knew nothing, a mystery within. I knew what she saw and heard only as feeling and when I was ill, only as feeling bad. With my child's imagination I thought she might be able to see and listen into the place inside me where fear and nightmares arose. Regardless of whether or not she could, her prescription of bed rest for most ailments salved that other place too because staying in bed at home brought more attention. Often my mother would sit with me while I ate my meal in bed and then because I did not read until the age of 11, she would read me stories and sing me songs at night to get to sleep.

As she examined me in my bed, Dr. Farmer peered through her glasses with great intensity. I was the whole focus of her attention. I gave back my full attention to her. How many times did I study that face! The soft skin of her cheeks covered with the light down of an elder, her finely defined nostrils, the thick grey eyebrows. It was a gentle intelligent face. Although she did not smile as she examined me, I noticed that she had what I would now identify as a look of profound interest and compassionate care accompanied by a sense of authority. As I said, she exuded trustworthiness. In the 1950s, someone with the title of doctor was understood to have an humanitarian calling. Dr. Farmer fit with that understanding. She made me feel I was a person worthy of attention.

For me the image of the profession changed in the early 1960s when Dr. Farmer retired and I was forced to go to a male pediatrician in town whose office was in a basement room in his house in a residential neighborhood. There were no enchanted rooms adjacent to the office, no image of the doctor as a child in his waiting area. He was a formal man in a coat and tie who regarded me as a collection of measurements and symptoms. His examination transformed my sense of my inner body from mystery to process and function. This was reinforced by his distant condescending manner which was characteristic of the paternalistic style of some doctors of the time. Nor did he have the penetrating gaze of Dr. Farmer. I remember him in the pantheon of my youth as the representative of the advancement of technological medicine and a new pharmacopeia. I do not recall him ever prescribing bed rest.

Much of the difference of the two may have been a difference of temperament, and of course, my response to the two doctors may have had much to do with the difference of my age and consciousness when I saw each, but for me, looking back, it seems to have been a moment of transition in the professional practice of medicine. Yet whatever the nature of the difference, to me it is most significant that the new doctor never made house calls to our house. The doctor bag that inspired my treasure chest was the legacy of Dr. Farmer exclusively. I wanted my chest to acquire the magic, enchantment and healing power that I associated with Dr. Farmer. Now after nine years I recognize in the response of others that it has achieved some of what I had hoped.

Gradually my treasure chest acquired magical instruments and objects that could bring "healing." I have a few hats in the chest with which I change character. There is the Irish cap worn by Rupert, the chimney sweep, about whom I will have more to say later. Rupert also keeps his magic brush on the shelf in the chest. There is the baker's hat worn by Francois, who takes all of a patient's bad feelings and transforms them into a delicious sourdough bread or if they are about to be discharged, bakes a cake to celebrate the sweet moment. And there is a Turkish red skullcap with small mirrors sewn into the fabric and embroidered with gold embroidery. This is sometimes (but not always) used for wizardry such as that associated with the Music of the Spheres and the playing of the music of healing which will also be discussed later. For that music, I carry a brass Tibetan singing bowl and wooden wand in the chest. There is also a hollow blue glass ball that holds "Moon Powder." When a light is shown through the ball onto the patient, the curative powers of "Moon Powder" are activated. Of course, the therapeutic, pharmacological, and healthful benefits of these instruments in the

Treasure Chest can only be accessed and activated by one who is licensed to wear a red nose and inspired to behave accordingly.

"Moon Powder" magically appeared in my magical pharmacopeia through the compounding of two potencies. In a magical pharmacopeia imaginative creations are concocted to meet, enliven and reinforce imagination in the patient. Medications are not fantasized into existence and distributed to patients to bamboozle them. I have no aspirations to the role of the charlatans of the old traveling medicine shows who hawked and peddled snake oil to the gullible. Instead I offer patients gifts of a magical repertoire in which imaginative creations acknowledge and serve the essence and source of being. Henri Corbin, a Sufi scholar, used the term imaginal to refer to imaginations that expand into awareness of the essence and source of being. Following in that vein, I liken my magical pharmacopeia to poetry in which imagined creations are in service to the creative faculty by which consciousness opens to the depth and meaning of life.

The first potency in the compounding of Moon Powder is the magical influence of the moon upon imagination. Out in the vast reaches of space, the sun is a constant for us in our daily lives.

But the continually changing countenance of the moon stirs our imagination from an early age as the moon pulls on the tides and our blood. Even from an early age we think, "Something dramatic is happening out there in space." And mystery abides in the moon's changes. Yet when the moon turns its full face on us, it bestows on us a sense of intimacy. It is a paradox that ignites imagination that the moon communicates intimacy with the immensity of the cosmos.

The power of light is the second potency compounded in Moon Powder. There are, of course, many ways of envisioning the power of light. Here is how light became part of my pharmacopeia in hospital rooms.

One day, early in my first year in the hospital when each day seemed to suggest new possibilities for developing my work, an eighteen-month-old boy came crying into the Emergency Room of the hospital with his grandmother. He had hit his head on a kitchen cupboard while she was taking care of him and had a laceration on his forehead. Approaching them as they were ushered into a room, I found my attention seemed to distract and calm him. I decided to stay with them in the hope that I might continue to hold his attention while the nurse technician took his vital signs.

As she placed the pulse-ox with its red light on his finger, the boy became intrigued with the red glow. Responding to his interest in the light, I pulled my mini-flashlight from the breast pocket of my lab coat and said, "You have a light and I have a light." I aimed the flashlight down at the mattress in front of the boy where it made a small disk of light on the white sheet. He grabbed to catch the disk of light; I moved it away. He tried again; I moved the disk before he could catch it. This happened several times as we improvised a game of catching the light. Finally I decided to rest the light in his open palm. He held the light in his hand and gazed at it. For both of us in the moment, there seemed to be an inexplicable sense of the tactility of light. By then the tech had recorded vital signs and the doctor came into the room to examine the contusion.

As I left the room the charge nurse at the nursing station said to me, "That worked," meaning from her point of view I had successfully helped to facilitate a hospital procedure. "That?..." I responded, making an association as I began to speak, "That was just a variation on one of the greatest clown entrees in circus history." I was referring to Emmett Kelly's famous clown entree in the center ring of Ringling Brothers Barnum and Bailey Circus, which I had the good fortune to witness as a child in the audience at the circus. Emmett Kelly was then the master clown of the circus. His character, Carpet the Tramp, was a hobo dressed in a dilapidated hat and ragged jacket and pants, with the make-up suggestion of a scruffy beard setting off his bulbous nose. His clown entree was a solo act somewhere in the middle of the schedule of acts in the center ring. It began with the hobo sweeping up the center ring with a broom like a janitor sweeping dust. He came to a pool of light which he tried to sweep away. It grew smaller, but it eluded him and refused to disappear. When he tried to leave the ring, it pursued him. In reports I have read of the act he finally succeeded in sweeping the light under the circus ground cloth. The way I remember what happened in the act I saw, however, was different. As I remember it, at the end, the hobo got a large dust pan and swept the light into the dust pan with his broom, lifted the pan slowly and finally dropped it into an oil drum at the edge of the ring which was placed there to receive deposits after animal acts. As the pool of light vanished, momentarily the circus went dark. It was a simple act with powerful impact. The audience sat hushed in silence at the end of it. For they realized that Carpet the Tramp had mastered the forces of light and dark and by implication he had taken charge of the mysteries of life and death. There in an emergency room of the hospital a child and I had discovered a remote connection with Carpet the Tramp and a bit of the mystery and power of the manipulation of light.

So Moon Powder was a compounding of two potencies: the power of the Moon and the power of light.

Dr. Merryandrew: When Moon Powder was first used in the Emergency Room of the hospital, the doctor in the room brushed it off in disbelief, "Moon Powder?" But she did not know the transformational properties of Moon Powder. If the moon can change its shape in space each day over the course of a month, surely its powder has the power to change things on earth.

Let me tell you about Moon Powder. Moon Powder is collected from the slanted rays of moonlight coming through the trees in a forest in the time of the full moon. It is best collected in a crockery jar, which is held open in the forest to receive the moonlight and then sealed tightly with a lid so no light escapes. The light must be held in the totally dark sealed container until the time of the new moon when the sky is dark. Then it can be released into a globe placed over the opening of the container when the lid is removed. The light that has been contained and held for 14 days becomes powder in the globe.

Moon Powder is activated by shining a light through the globe and shaking the globe over the patient to be treated. It is best to turn the overhead lighting off in the room, leaving only the computer light and the light over the side counter in the room. Just as the moon changes each day of the month in the night sky, Moon Powder has the gift of change and it can change disease into health and pain into comfort.

I have used Moon Powder to positive effect in several instances. In one instance for example, a 6-year-old boy came to the Emergency Room with his grandmother. He complained of leg pain after jumping from a height. I told him that I needed to treat his pain with Moon Powder and proceeded to tell him the story of Moon Powder. He listened with wide-eyed attentiveness to how Moon Powder is gathered while his grandmother chuckled with each twist in my tale. When I finished shining the light of Moon Powder over him, the patient lowered himself off the Emergency Room bed and walked easily with no evident pain in his legs to the door of the room and back again to his bed. The Physician's Assistant reported to me later that the boy had told her, "That clown cured me."

This is but one example of many that attest to the efficacy of Moon Powder.

It might be believed that the efficacy of Moon Powder requires that the patient be willing to be cured and that doubt of its potency would interfere with its effectiveness. But a stance of ironic disbelief seems only to add to the benefit of treatment. One day I attended to a twelve-year-old patient who kept rolling her eyes as I told her the story of Moon Powder. She laughed in disbelief, forgetting in the instant the intestinal pain she had complained of when she came to the Emergency Department. Her mother and father laughed too.

Although there was an obvious difference in response, I do not honestly think that the 6-year-old child believed that I had cured him with Moon Powder anymore than the twelve-year-old did. So I have asked myself questions about what might be similar in their reactions and what was different because I have felt their responses give insight into the nature of my medical clowning in general. Most importantly, in stepping into the room and engaging a child in a moment of imagination, I establish a relationship with the child on the plane of play, which is familiar and comfortable to the child. To express that in another way, I am giving the child some caring and loving attention that carries no threat. Moreover, as is evident in both examples I have given, I immediately shift the focus of the child's imagination away from the pain that brought him or her into the ED. Even adults know that kind of shift has immediate salutary benefits. Whether a child plays along with my imagination or laughs it off, the dark heavy shroud over pain or illness lifts and the possibility of light and lightness enters the room for the child. Somehow in the moment, there is a palpable relief, which, you might say, is not a bad ministration for pain or illness.

If there was an underlying difference between the responses of the 6-year-old boy and the 12-year-old girl to being treated with Moon Powder other than the expressed difference, I cannot be sure, but I can imagine. For the 6-year-old, the initial complaint may have been inspired by fear and imagination. He may have done something while playing that startled him, gave him an immediate hurt that became enlarged by his imagination. Then you might say, Moon Powder transformed that imagination by substitution or "sympathetic magic." I am more inclined to acknowledge the physical foundation for the 12-year-old girl's initial complaint. She found herself in the hospital because of a sharp abdominal pain. But as we all have experienced, many acute abdominal pains that are not severe resolve themselves with time. Often they are transient experiences of our digestive system. This may have been the case for the 12-year-old. To give myself a bit of credit here, the laughter, which flexes and releases the abdominal muscles, may have accelerated the relief, also a kind of sympathetic magic. So I persist with my tales and folly.

Last but not least, my "treasure box" medical case has become my means for transporting Jamie, my child, assistant, diagnostician and alter ego.

Chapter Two

Listen!

Standing before this door to begin my clown rounds on this day, I can still access the feelings of trepidation with which I stood before this door on my first day. As I have already mentioned, I was startled to be here. I wondered anxiously how and why I had gotten to that moment and what I thought I might do after I entered the room. Fortunately, I did not linger outside the door too long. I pulled myself up in my shoes, opened the door and delivered my doggerel of introduction with my best representation of confidence.

In all honesty to this day, I still feel some degree of that same trepidation each time I prepare to knock at a door and enter a patient room. As many times now as I have gone into hospital rooms, it is still the case that I hesitate. I still do not know whom or what I will encounter. Consequently, I do not know what I will find in myself to meet the circumstances in the room.

Seasoned by the years of working, of course, I have learned to anticipate certain characteristics of illnesses from the brief descriptions of diagnoses in the census. What I have learned in that regard, however, matters little to alleviate the anxiety of anticipation since my concern is to encounter patients, not diseases, and for each patient the characteristics of an illness can manifest so differently. Besides, the personalities and the life circumstances of patients are not noted in the census descriptions. Unless I have come to know a patient with a chronic disease, who has to be hospitalized frequently, I do not know whom I am about to meet, nor do I know whom or what I will encounter among the patient's family and friends. Holding too many variables and possibilities, I cannot be entirely prepared for the circumstances I will encounter. I have watched doctors and nurses I admire stride into a room with the great confidence of their expertise. But for my part, I go to the door more humbly, for I have to allow the circumstances to evoke the performance.

In the months after I started work at the hospital, I prompted myself into a representation of boldness hoping I would take on the pretended confidence. But I was honest with myself about what I could sustain and whether or not something I did in one room could carry over to others. Then I came home each day from the hospital and wrote notes about what I had done in each patient's room. I noted what was successful and what failed. I engaged myself in a dialogue about my role and responsibility as a clown in the realm of healthcare. As I started out, I wrote to a former student of mine about my inner debate:

> Since I am on my own in this and this is such different kind of work from any performing I have ever done, I am all in a dither about it. I worry about costume. Will it be acceptable to people without being scary to children who might be afraid of clowns? What can I do as a performer in a hospital room? Who am I performing for, child patients or their parents or the hospital staff or all? How do I improvise when I am given nothing to go on? Should I be myself in costume or should I have a strong clown character and persona? If I hit it too hard, I may feel good, but will I really be reaching patients?

As I walked my dog in the afternoon or evening, I would reflect on the day, evaluate my experience and consider corrections where I felt correction was needed. Here from my notes are questions I raised for myself as a performer in the hospital setting.

> 4/11/2011: As I walked with Misha in the afternoon, I realized I have gone into the hospital with the desire to entertain or, maybe even worse, to please. Such a desire in this case is not a practical objective because I haven't a clue what would please in the situation. Anyway, there are too many changing variables to try to please. On what basis might I please? Bad objective? To amuse might be an objective if I were ready to draw all the attention to myself, but I am not certain that is my goal. I want to meet what is there in the children, parents and staff. I am not ready to play all bravado. I am thinking I want a subtler clown…

In the evolution of the work with patients, those early questions I posed for myself kept recurring. Looking back at my questioning, I see

I focused on two different aspects of the work. Separating the two is, to be sure, an analytical construct. In practice these different ways of considering what I was doing were not separable, but I find it helpful to articulate them as separate areas of concern.

First of all, as a performer I kept questioning the aesthetic quality of what I was doing. What do I mean by that? In simple terms, I kept asking myself if what I was doing for patients and others in the room was worthy of their attention. As I created performances in the rooms, I held myself to a creative aesthetic. Was what I was doing engaging? Was there rhythmic variation in a performance? How could I use movement, gesture, speech, and music? How could I use story and poetry? How could I use props? How could I use puppets? How could I invite patients, family members, nurses, and doctors into a performance without shattering the imaginary frame? How could I use different characterizations and change characters in the rooms?

The other aspect of my work about which my questioning circled was the social or ethical nature of it. The fundamental concern underlying such questions is how am I serving patients in the hospital? I ask myself am I entertaining? Am I distracting from pain or fear? Am I alleviating parental anxiety? Am I offering patients an opportunity to feel more like themselves, instead of being defined by disease? Can everyone in the room relax with me present? Is there some magic at moments with patients when something unexpected happens? Are there moments that touch the heart? What do those moments suggest? Are there moments that inspire? What do those moments suggest? Am I affirming for the patients? Do I offer some ease in a time of disease? All such questions subsumed in one, that one question: Am I helpful in some way to the patient, family and medical staff?

The way in which I have tried to live into questions and maybe, through them into answers is to listen. In the aesthetic, I try to attune my third ear, or inner sensitivity, to be alert to rhythm and balance. Sometimes, the narrative flow needs the break of a digression, something to slow time and to give more time for the patient to enter imaginatively into the narrative with me. Sometimes, I feel the soothing rhythm of repetition will gently build a feeling of expectation to be fulfilled or broken for effect. Some interaction seems to need the elevation of a song. At other times, I feel a song provides relief from a surfeit of intensity or fixation. In the ethical, I try to attune my inner ear to the tenor and tension in the room, to signs of fear, fatigue, anxiety, loneliness, welcome, ease, or even joyfulness. I listen to the interaction of family with the patient, patient with nurses and doctors, family with nurses and doctors. I hear the noise of television, cellphones, iPads, computers, monitors, and IV drips as external static that plays against the inner music in a patient and in us all.

I try to stay especially attuned to my own impact on the people and circumstances in the room. That can often be a difficult assessment because patients responses are not so easy to read. They are coping with pain and medications that often make them tired or sometimes, overly stimulated. Because they frequently have intrusive visitors, they are often wary of anyone, even someone with the best intentions. Sometimes when they shy away from the clown with the red nose and lab coat, they delight to meet my miniature in my marionette. At other times, I have discovered patients who are so at ease with me that I am surprised and disarmed that they become fearful and rejecting when I introduce them to my marionette. Sometimes, I have been incorporated into the interactions within a family or the interactions between patients and nurses and doctors. I have been enlisted in alignments that are there or have formed for unknown reasons before I entered the room.

In a hospital room, where relationships and reactions are generally intensified because of the circumstances of disease and injury, what almost instantaneous assumptions are made about me can be startling and play against my efforts to attune to the undertones for feelings of wellness in the room. Sometimes, to be sure, I become self-consciously concerned with how I have become embroiled in dynamics in the room for which I have sparse understanding. I have been enlisted by teenagers in their conflicts with mom. Likewise, I have been recruited by a parent for support against a rebellious child. Sometimes patients even try to align me with them against the doctors who have seen them or against the treatment they are being given. I do my best diplomatically to negotiate my way out of all such problematic alignments. Yet I have to recognize that they are just extreme instances of the common sense truth that I cannot walk into a hospital room, introduce myself and have patients take me at face value. I have to accept that with my clown nose, my lab coat and my treasure chest, I am a symbol entering the room.

I am not just another person; I am a character, a clown. Like all symbols, I evoke associations, expectations, thoughts, and emotions. Notions of who I am are projected on me before I have an opportunity to identify Dr. Merryandrew with a story, a characterization, or a song of my own.

I mentioned earlier that I deliberately created an ambiguity when I was costuming Dr. Merryandrew. Initially the ambiguity was intended simply to establish Dr. Merryandrew as a clown doctor or doctor clown. I hoped to communicate immediately, visually that I was indeed a clown, but a clown concerned with the art of healing. I wanted to dissuade anyone from thinking I was a prankster clown, a juggler, a bumbling fool, or a slapstick trickster out to make everyone else feel foolish. I find, however, the ambiguous image I present often evokes response that does not take into account the paradox implicit in the ambiguity. Some just see the red nose. With them, I always feel awkward when I have to apologize for not making balloon sculptures, even though latex is forbidden around patients. On the other hand, with those for whom my lab coat seems to dominate the impression they have of me who sometimes embarrassingly assume I am their doctor and immediately start to provide me with a full medical history of their child's condition, I have to make an awkward apology for the misunderstanding.

In the early days of my first year in the hospital, I wrote myself a prospectus for the work. In it I tried to tie what I hoped to do into how I understood the language of medical tradition in particular Hippocrates and the Hippocratic Oath. At that time I wrote myself a "mission statement" for my work.

> Mission Statement: The mission of a clown doctor is to help patients restore themselves to a sense of well-being through playful interaction. The guiding principles of the work are the fundamental principles of the Hippocratic Oath: to benefit all patients by the best possible means available, to show compassion and to do no harm. A clown doctor works with the resources of humor and imagination.

I understood the purpose of a mission statement was to present the nature of the work as directly and simply as possible without evaluative implication. I wrote my own mission statement to provide a simple touchstone to remind myself of what motivated me to begin to serve as a medical clown. Whatever I learned as I went along about doing the work of a medical clown, I did not want to forget the point at which I started. To some degree, I would say that I have never needed to go beyond what I set down then. I have, however, learned much regarding the "best possible means" with which to do the work, of course, taking into account my own capabilities as a performer and person. As for "compassion," one does not learn more about compassion. One is either compassionate or not. But certainly through the experience I have had, I have had the opportunity to extend the range of my compassion and to explore different ways of showing my concern for others. Since I do not place IV lines, do no surgeries, do not administer medications, the risks of my doing harm are not physical or biochemical. But I must be cautious, nonetheless, not to exacerbate feelings of fear or stress for anyone. If a patient turns away when I poke my head in the room, I exit with an apology. If a child shows some anxiety during anything I am doing, I simply stop, ask if he or she would like me to stop, and quickly fold up if so requested. It would be inappropriate for me to make demands of patients. On the contrary, my hope is to offer patients release and relief and to direct them through whatever art I have toward their own inner capacity for a sense of well-being, instead of toward disease.

One slow day in the Pediatric emergency department, in order to relieve the pressure on the adult emergency department, we took a thirty-two year-old patient who had an uncomplicated complaint. While he was waiting for the result of a test sent to the lab, I went to visit him. We had a relaxed human-to-human exchange, nothing more. Later his nurse told me, he reported to her that he enjoyed my visit. He told her I have a good bedside manner. She and I laughed about that and I jokingly remarked, "That's what my work is all about, bedside manner." Yes, it is a joke because I like to think I offer a bit more than that. But I do not mind the characterization at all. As I have indicated earlier in my mention of my own pediatrician, Dr. Elsa Farmer, it is no denigration of the value of my work to compare it with the fine bedside manner of a good doctor.

Recently after years in the hospital, I read Nortin Hadler's wonderful book, *By the Bedside of the Patient: Lessons for the Twenty-First-Century Physician.* Had it been published before I started at the hospital instead of many years after, I might have phrased my mission statement in relation to something I learned about in Hadler's book. Instead of taking as my guide the principles of Hippocrates, I think I might have done well to adopt "The Morning Prayer of the Physician," as my model. In its known form, Hadler reports, the prayer was printed in 1793, as written by a German Physician named Marcus Herz, who was a student of Immanuel Kant and physician to Moses Mendelssohn, though it has been attributed to two philosopher/physicians, Moses Maimonides in the 12th century and Avicenna in the 11th century. Hadler gives the prayer in his book.

The Morning Prayer of the Physician

> O God, let my mind be ever clear and
>   enlightened.
> By the bedside of the patient let no alien
>   thought deflect it.
> Let everything that experience and
>   scholarship have
> taught it be present in it and hinder it
>   not in its tranquil work.
> For great and noble are those scientific
>   judgments that serve
> the purpose of preserving the health
>   and lives of Thy creatures.

Keep far from me the delusion that I can
accomplish all things.
Give me the strength, the will, and the
opportunity
to amplify my knowledge more and
more.
Today I can disclose things in my
knowledge which yesterday
I would not yet have dreamt of for the
art is great,
but the human mind presses on untir-
ingly.

In the patient let me ever see only the
man.
Thou, All-Bountiful One, hast chosen
me to watch over
the life and death of Thy creatures.
I prepare myself now for my calling.
Stand Thou by me in this great task, so
that it may prosper.
For without Thine aid man prospers
not even in the smallest things.[1]

Needless to say, my resources are not the
scientific judgments to which the prayer refers.
Nor am I entitled to suggest that what I do

directly preserves health and life. My resources are art dedicated to help patients access their own inner sense of well-being. But the responsibility and humility expressed in the prayer are qualities toward which I strive. When I say to myself before entering patient rooms, "It's not about you. Listen!" I feel that responsibility and humility.

In that regard, I recognize that behind what I have identified as my aesthetic and ethical questions about this work, I hold the spiritual question to be asked of any work hoping to serve in the world. In all such work the most fundamental way of asking the question I am referring to as the spiritual question is, "How can I serve?" For me in my own work in the hospital, I find the way to pose the spiritual question to myself is by asking, "Is this a meaningful practice?" Without the pretension of equivalence, I can set my own query beside that of some physicians who question the appropriateness of offering patients certain procedures. For instance in the literature regarding terminal illness, some physicians question offering patients procedures simply because they are available though there is no claim of efficacy. In *By the Bedside of the Patient*, Hadler raises questions regarding the appropriateness of certain cardiac procedures and certain treatments in his own field of rheumatology. He recommends that clinical procedures come under efficacy review and that the effectiveness of such procedures be determined and communicated in plain language so that patients can weigh risks against benefits. Similar concern was raised by one of our Intensive Care doctors in pediatrics in a conversation I had with him. From pediatric intensive care, most patients recover and get to go home in a relatively short time. In adult intensive care units, however, he felt it was a disturbing statistic that the survival rates were not much better than 20%. Too many patients did not recover from interventions provided. He expressed futility with that figure. As I write, too, I know that questions of this sort are circulating in intensive care units around the country during the COVID19 pandemic. Doctors are finding it difficult not to be able to offer patients more effective treatment. It challenges the meaningfulness of the physicians presence. I understand that there are those who recognize that in the final determination, what they can offer as physicians, confronting a disease for which there is too little understanding, is no more, but certainly no less, than the presence of a caring human being at the bedside of the patient.

For myself and my work, however, I do have to qualify that when I ask if my practice is meaningful, the spiritual question I am asking is different than that of the physician. My own question does not question the efficacy of treatment. I am not asking in order to evaluate outcome or probability of outcome. The implicit assumptions of the question of usefulness are not appropriate to the intentions of my own work with patients. I am not oriented to cause and effect assessment of treatment or to outcome of treatment, at all. For I do not define what I do as therapy. I ponder the meaningfulness of the work, rather, in relation to the existential experience of illness. Since we all experience illness as a part of being alive, we cannot rid ourselves of it the way treatment or therapy can alleviate the symptoms of disease nor can we understand moments of illness as moments outside of life. Though uncomfortable, they are necessary experiences of life. How we make meaning of them; how we find meaning in them, is my concern. When I ask if my practice is meaningful, I am asking if it serves in patients' efforts to make meaning of their experiences of illness and time in the hospital.

For reasons I will elaborate later, I started at the hospital with the understanding that illness and hospitalization are liminal experiences. Let me clarify what I mean by that. The term liminal, as I understand it, was introduced by the anthropologist, Arnold van Gennep, writing about rites of passage in 1960 and then expanded upon by Victor Turner in his anthropological studies, to refer to events that can be characterized as in-between, marginal or transitional states on the threshold of some moment of significant transition in life. They are experienced as moments out of time. Van Gennep demonstrated that rites of passage go through three phases: separation, transition or liminal, and aggregation. For example, in an initiation ritual, novitiates are symbolically removed from their status in society. They experience a period of isolation which is understood as being in-between worlds, between before and after, between childhood and adulthood. Then they are re-incorporated into a new status in society. In his seminal book, entitled *The Ritual Process*, Turner elaborated on the profound significance of the liminal period.

> The attributes of liminality or of liminal personae ('threshold people') are necessarily ambiguous, since this condition and these persons elude or slip

through the network of classifications that normally locate states and positions in cultural space. Liminal entities are neither here nor there; they are betwixt and between the positions assigned and arrayed by law, custom, convention, and ceremonial. As such their ambiguous and indeterminate attributes are expressed by a rich variety of symbols in the many societies that ritualize social and cultural transitions. Thus, liminality is frequently likened to death, to being in the womb, to invisibility, to darkness, to bisexuality, to the wilderness, and to an eclipse of the sun or moon.[2]

In traditional societies, ritual clowns commonly inhabit realms of the liminal. In ceremonies and initiations, often they are masked and costumed to impersonate mythical beings half animal half human, ancestors or natural deities. They get their powers and magic from the source of the sacred.

Our secular society and culture in comparison with traditional societies, however, has a paucity of rites of passage. When I taught literature for seven years in a private high school, I was concerned that while most high school age students in our society are going through a major transitional period of their lives, they are offered no rite of passage, no ritual of initiation to guide their successful transition toward commitment and responsibility in adulthood. Consequently, because I had the good fortune to work with the students in the school over all of their four years of high school, I chose to structure what I taught and how I taught as initiatory experience. I recognize some of my understanding of adolescence from my years of teaching carries over to my sense of illness as liminal. Adolescents are full of paradox and ambiguity. They have a strong feeling for the urgency of their moment of life while they seem to think of themselves as immortal, living in an eternity of time. They do not live in the measured time of yesterdays progressing toward tomorrow; they do not take into account the memories of the past as they make plans for the future. For them, time does not creep "in this petty pace from day to day." Rather time rolls in waves with peaks of outward passion and troughs of inwardness and withdrawal. Sometimes they exert intense effort to meet the moment, only later to slip into stolid indolence. Yet all life's moments are imbued with great significance. Patients often take up their illnesses with a similar intensity. They can swing between extremes of now and eternity, between moments in which they are alert to the fullness of life and moments of emptiness, fatigue and resignation. They sit in the threshold of time where all life's moments are filled with significance.

I feel, however, because of the absence of ceremonial attention to transitional experience in society that might contribute to understanding illness as liminal, illness is experienced without that understanding, yet existentially experienced as liminal nonetheless. For illness in general, and especially illness that requires hospitalization, occurs in phases similar to the three phases of rites of passage. First it removes us from the ordinary flow of our lives to a place of isolation. Then we find ourselves in a state of being betwixt and between, neither here nor there. We may have intimations of our own mortality or actually come near to dying. We may feel the sun of our lives eclipsed. We may also glimpse in the stillness of the hour a sense of the eternal or the holy, of destiny or meaning. Finally as we recover, we return to family and community, and not infrequently after serious illness, we are changed and our alignments in our families and communities are changed. With this sense of illness as liminal with which I started this work and which I found to be reinforced in my day to day practice, I began to formulate the spiritual question of the meaningfulness of what I do. Could what I offer help patients find richer meaning in their lives during the transitional experience of illness and hospitalization?

Aesthetic, moral and spiritual questions, these are the questions I hold within myself as I stand poised to enter at the door of each patient room; as I pause and tell myself: "It's not about you. Listen!" It is a moment fraught with awe and humility. I am aware that what I do entails responsibility and mystery. Though I trade in levity, I do not take the work lightly. After all, I engage in this work to be of service to fellow human beings in God's Hotel. (Hotel Dieu was the term used in the Middle Ages to refer to a place at a monastery where the ill went for care.)

Chapter Three

The Shield of Light

A word about method and structure is perhaps in order at this point. I intended from the outset of this book to try to bring you, Readers, along as I round on a characteristic day in the hospital, this day. My objective is simultaneously to make a book and a day. If you have come this far with me, however, you may be wondering if that was ever in the plan despite the early indication to that effect. I am aware that it may seem that I have been distracted from my original purpose. But in apology and, I suppose, as excuse for the seeming meandering nature of my narrative so far, I offer that I have engaged this project with a Shandian sensibility for the comic (that is in the spirit of *Tristram Shandy*, Laurence Sterne's 18th century comic novel), to proceed through a series of diversions (rather than consistently direct pursuit) and only later to discover that what seemed the most roundabout route was, to the contrary, a felicitous path to the intended end. As a lover of the silent clowns of the great film era before talkies, of Charlie Chaplin, Buster Keaton, Harold Lloyd, Harry Langdon, Stan Laurel and Oliver Hardy and the rest, at least, I feel I am in the good company of those who went roundabout to get where they were going. To the tragic sense of life belong narratives that follow the straight and narrow course of purpose, passion and perspective. In the spirit of the comic vision, I will make my way, occasionally veering here and there, yet somehow covering the intended trajectory and hopefully arriving at my destination with a sense of recognition and acceptance for the course I have taken to get there. For now, if that can be accepted, I shall make haste slowly to recover in this narrative a sense of the day.

Here we are still outside the very first door where we began. We are poised to listen. Since I am not authorized to view charts, before entering a room, I take a careful look at what information the census can provide. A census is not a very informative document. It has about as much information about patients as an itinerary of a grand tour has about European cities. Sometimes

I feel like the village idiot poring over the census trying to interpret what is there. It is a bit like trying to get a feeling for those cities from the names and dates written on the itinerary, but I try to make the most of what is given. It is a great advantage to know a patient's name before entering a room. Most of the time the census will provide both the first and last name. When first names are left off, it is less helpful. Nevertheless, because I seldom get a name before I enter an emergency room, I have become comfortable with the blunt request to be told a name. The census does provide age, abbreviated diagnosis, number of days patients have been hospitalized, dates of birth, and expected dates of discharge.

As I have said, I do not enter rooms to engage with diseases, but the diagnoses help me anticipate the patients' conditions. The number of days a patient has been hospitalized can also suggest the patient's condition. There is a rhythm to hospital stays. As I have already mentioned in the last chapter, that rhythm is comparable to the rhythm of other liminal experiences. First or second days have the greatest intensity, which I would characterize by qualities of openness and supplication. Generally, last days are characterized by the anticipation of returning to the social context from which the patient has been removed.

Of course, with children age listed on the census is a helpful indicator of expected developmental level, but developmental delay is not infrequent, so age can often be an unreliable reading. Occasionally, date of birth listed on the census alerts me to past or anticipated celebrations. Although I know little of astrology, sometimes I amuse myself by guessing at personality from zodiacal signs. For me, however, that is just a game. When I am in an adult unit, I do find age provides a gross indication of a patient's locus in the seasons of life.

Though I try to make the most of the little information it provides, there are days when I can stare at the census blankly, hoping to read some insight in the runes, yet finding nothing there. Then I begin my rounds feeling empty handed, except for my mantra, "Listen!"

Empty handed is really not a bad place to start. Just as my mantra tells me to empty myself of myself as I enter the room, getting nothing from the census allows me to encounter patients without preconceptions about them. So that is where I will begin on this day to enter this and other rooms.

Dr. Merryandrew: Good Morning. I am Dr. Merrryandrew
    I am the doctor who treats your ills
    with tales and folly instead of pills.
I stopped in to see if I could do something for you today.

While introducing myself and just after, I wait for some indication that I am invited to continue. That indication may come as a smile, leaning back on the pillows in the bed and setting a cellphone down, turning off the television, or a word like "Okay," "Sure," or "Yeah." Sometimes if the patient hesitates before responding, I jump in with a quick suggestion of what I feel I can offer in the moment. A spontaneous choice to act may be the best way for me to meet the patient. Though it might seem that such a spontaneous choice is arbitrary, there are indefinable elements in the room that do influence me in the moment – the sense of the patient's mood, a shift of posture or expression; a look or gesture from a patient; a toy, blanket, personal pillow, stuffed animal, or book in the bed or on the tray beside the bed. Anything unique to the patient, can give me a hint of something to which to respond. Or I may try to deflect a rejection before it comes by asking, "What's going on for you today?" All I am looking for is an opening in the channel of communication. For instance, today the girl and her mother stop playing the board game with which they are engaged, sit up instead of hunching over the bed tray that holds the playing board and smile a warm greeting.

Because the patient is a teenager and alert enough to follow a longish routine, I suggest I would like to offer her protection. Jokingly I reassure her mother that I am not selling insurance; not to worry.

Dr. Merryandrew: But I have to test you to see if you are a candidate for protection. How are you at tests?

So begins my introduction to a routine I call the Shield of Light. This routine evolved as the very first way I came to address patients' sense that their sun has been eclipsed and they have been cast into the umbrage of disease. I never intended more by declaring that I was going to test the patient than to create an atmosphere of mock seriousness. But I have had times that I have reconsidered that way of starting. Sometimes I fear it seems all too "teacherly" and might evoke too strong an association with school. Though I have to admit there is something of the scholar/ teacher in Dr. Merryandrew, as there was more than a little of the performer in my manner of teaching. For from the scholarly side of his character, Dr. Merryandrew gets his posture of authority. Conversely, when I was a high school teacher, I tried to bring lightness and passion to teaching by borrowing from all my years as a professional performer.

In truth, over time I have come to recognize that patients are way ahead of me in understanding my mock examination. They do not make an association with school or medical exams at all or at least for not longer than a flash. Instead they take up the question about taking tests with a twist. I have never had a patient tell me that she is not good at test taking. The worst that I ever hear a patient claim is that she is "so-so" at taking tests. It may be true that all the patients I see are good test takers, but it seems to me rather that they have heard the question as an opportunity to give a self-assessment, and answer a more general and global question about themselves, as if I had asked, "How do you assess yourself and your competence?" They are very ready to answer, "I'm good." So what I get in response to my "too teacherly question" is something better than I deserve to expect; patients assess themselves as competent and "good." This is a significant shift from feeling bad and bad about themselves to feeling good about themselves and how they function in the world. It is, to be sure, a response evoked in the moment and a small gesture, but a gesture, nevertheless, of self-respect and self-confidence. That makes my work easy; we are on the way together down the comic road that is always the way of affirmation. The sun begins to slip from the shadow that hid its brightness.

Reassured that we are together, I pull the penlight from my chest pocket, turn it on pointing down toward the bed and request that the patient tell me what he or she sees as I send the light around the patient's body. Coming full circle with the light, I ask,

Dr. Merryandrew: Well, what did you see?

This is, of course, meant to elicit any number of possible wrong answers: "I didn't see anything." "I saw a light going in a circle." "I saw the bed." Sometimes I will even elicit a suggestion from a parent or friend in the room as if I am allowing the patient to have some help. Of course, all the answers are literally correct in terms of what the patient perceived visually as I moved the light in a circle. But this is the moment where perceivable truth and imagined reality part ways. I pull a kazoo from my coat pocket and say through the kazoo so that the sound vibrates enough to be almost unrecognizable as words, but has a distinctly recognizable inflection pattern,

Dr. Merryandrew: You didn't see it, Stephanie. You didn't see it.

Then with the kazoo out of my mouth and back in my pocket, I say in my own voice,

Dr. Merryandrew: I'll have to show you.

I start to create a wall in mimed movement around the patient following the path the light traveled. I never need to go very far along the circle to create the image.

Dr. Merryandrew: See. I created a shield of light around you. I promised you protection. I circled you with light for protection.

Marcel Marceau used to say that "Mime takes the visible and makes it invisible and takes the invisible and makes it visible." That is what I attempt to do with a few practiced gestures that create the shield of light. I want to make visible an invisible shield of light around the patient as an enveloping force field.

Dr. Merryandrew: It goes up to the ceiling, down to the floor, all around you.

As I move along the surface with my hands, the shield of light becomes very real to me, as I hope it will for the patient. I make a distinction between this palpable reality and phantasmal imagination. If it were illusion, I would simply be acting "as if" it were there. Initially, of course, that was how it was and how it can be at times even now. But, more often now, the "as if" becomes subsumed in the relational reality developing between the patient and me. In that context, the shield becomes a lighted and enlivening palpable reality. It takes on a tensile substantiality.

Experiencing the tensile space between people was part of my acting training. There is a well-known acting exercise known as the "Mirror Exercise," which was written up in the American bible of improvisational theater, *Improvisation for the Theater* by Viola Spolin, the teacher who originated the idea of training actors with theater games. The basic mirror exercise is very simple.

When I was teaching mime and theater, I modified it to make it just as simple as it could get. I would ask two students to face each other. One student would initiate movement and one would mirror the other. I always started this exercise by asking the students to place their hands opposite each other in the air but not touching. The game was to see if the pair could move their hands in such a way that someone watching could not tell who was initiating and who was mirroring. They learned very quickly that the mirror could not watch the initiator's hands. They could only succeed by looking into each other's eyes and "feeling" the movement. Occasionally, students would remark as they were doing this exercise, "It tickles." They could feel tensile communication on their palms.

In the early 1970s, Paul Sills, developed a delightful performance piece from the mirror exercise. Paul Sills was one of Viola Spolin's sons. He started a theater company that developed stage performances from the improvisational theater games of his mother. In 1970, "Story Theater," a stage performance directed by Sills and adapted from Grimm Brothers' Fairytales and Aesop's Fables, was a popular Off-Broadway production based on these improvisations. The shortest story in the production was about two crows trying to open a mussel shell. There are very few lines in the text. The impact of the performance came from the movement of the actors portraying the crows. They both wore baseball hats with yellow visors as bills. By moving their heads, stopping, tilting, turning toward another direction, up, down, right, left, diagonal, they mimicked the movement and relation of two birds sitting on a limb. As in the mirror exercise, the exact moves of the actors were not choreographed. The improvisational nature of the movement kept the sense of spontaneity. For the audience, the delight of the performance was to feel the dynamic tension spanning the space between the two crows, exposing the relation. Later when I became a performer, I cultivated in myself the capacity to stay alert to that tension in the space between people. It is that kind of tensile substance that I experience at the bedside of the patient.

Of course, I am also aware that the connection between people which is felt to have a tensile reality may facilitate substantive exchange. In my theater experience, I have seen that sometimes meaningful subconscious communication occurs through this space. On the simplest level, we all probably experience this when we turn to look at someone across a room and realize that person has been looking at us for some time in order to get our attention. On a more mysterious level, when I have been teaching students who felt "tickled" in the mirror exercise, I have taken the occasion to up the ante with a different but related exercise that I myself experienced as a student. I sat one student in a chair and asked the other student to stand some distance behind the chair. The student in the chair was simply asked to sit silently and think whatever thoughts he or she wished, moving only to adjust for comfort. The student behind was asked to sense the communications coming from the thinker in the chair and, without reflection, to move interpretively to express the thoughts of the thinker. It was remarkable in these instances that other students watching the two were always able to observe when the interpreter was in connection with the thinker and when the interpreter slipped out of communication with the thinker. As I said, the communication was subconscious and there was no apprehensible content exchange, yet the communication was obvious to all. I will not say that I always achieve this level of communication as I create a shield of light around a patient, but I do not deny that at times such communication does occur in the tensile space between us.

Back to the Shield of Light.

Dr. Merryandrew: (Continuing in mime) Look, there's a door. (Unlocking the door with a mimed key from his right coat pocket) Here, hold this key. Don't lose it. (Stepping back) You see. I promised you protection. Now you have a Shield of Light around you for protection. (Miming an enclosure around him as he talks and gesturing in illustration of his words) You step inside, lock the door, you're safe. When the coast is clear, unlock the door, go out into the big world. It's a beautiful world out here. The sun is shining. Birds are flying. Fruit is growing on trees. But if the dark hand of evil comes over you. Back inside, lock the door, you're safe. A Shield of Light for protection.

You know what it's like?... It's like a wrinkle in time. You know about wrinkles in time? (Often patients say they saw the recent movie, "A Wrinkle in Time," but they do not remember exactly what it is. Or at least, they are not able to describe it.) I'll tell you. You know about time, right? We learn this in school. Time is like a line. (He stretches a mimed line between his hands with his fingers and holds the tension of the imaginary line in front of him. Then with the index and pointer finger of his right hand, he creates an image of walking a tightrope.) Here we are yesterday. Here we are today. And here we are tomorrow. We walk from yesterday to today toward tomorrow. We never get to tomorrow, do we? By the time we get there, it's always today, isn't it?

(Here he shifts scale and begins to walk as if he himself is walking along a mimed tightrope.) It's sort of like walking a tightrope… or a slack rope. Do you know what a slack rope is? You know what a tightrope is, right? It's really a wire that is straight across. A slack rope is a real rope that hangs down loosely and swings a little as you walk it. Of course, your weight pulls the rope down into a V-shape so you are walking up hill all the time. It's hard to walk it. You know how you learn? I'll tell you. Learn to fall down. That's what my teacher taught me, learn to fall down. If you learn to fall down, then you're not afraid to fall. Bam. You get up; keep walking. Bam. Get up; keep walking. Pretty soon the rope becomes a highway. It's the same with life really. Learn to fall down. Bam. Get back up. Pretty soon life's a highway… Now where was I? I got distracted… Oh yeah, I was talking about time.

Obviously, Dr. Merryandrew has not wandered from his intention at this point. Initially I did not make the claim of being "distracted." After awhile, however, the comment on learning to fall and getting back up in life seemed to me to have a homiletic tone that I wanted to cover quickly. So I allow a brake in the frame of the performance for a little self-mockery.

Dr. Merryandrew: (Gesturing to illustrate the words again) Every now and then this time line wraps around itself. It gets what we call a wrinkle. Step inside the wrinkle, you disappear because all time and no time is there. Step back out, you're on the highway. Inside, you disappear. Outside, you're on the highway. It's the same with your light shield. You can disappear inside your light shield for awhile. Step back out, you're on the highway. I've got a song about the wrinkle in time. You want to hear it?

To be clear, the following song is not my own composition. These are the first two verses of a song by the wonderful singer song-writer, Bob Zentz. The song has the title "A Wrinkle in Time."

Doctor Merryandrew:
   Wish I had a wrinkle in time,
   a place where I could go,
   an autumn mountain I could climb
   leave the rest of the world below.

   Wish I had a place to sing
   these secret songs of mine
   where all the joy that singing brings
   would be with me all the time.

(Chorus) I'd close my eyes one instant and be
  gone
open 'em wide and I'd be back again.
Rested and strong from my world inside
and I'd never tell a soul where I had been.

Wish I had a laughing place
when this old world gets me down
where sorrow never knew my face
and my dreams were all around.

Wish I had a place to lose
this everyday routine
to hide my sorrows and my blues
from the good times I have seen.

(Chorus) I'd close my eyes one instant and be
  gone
open 'em wide and I'd be back again
rested and strong from my world inside
and I'd never tell a soul where I had been.

Wish I had a wrinkle in time...[3]

Bob Zentz writes in liner notes for "Wrinkle in Time" that the idea for the song came from reading the book, *A Wrinkle in Time,* by Madeleine

L'Engle, which happened to be made into a movie around the time I was beginning work in the hospital. He explains in liner notes for his album, *Beaucatcher Farewell,*

> The author expresses a concept of Time in which Time is not a straight line but a wrinkled one… It came to me one good day that, if we could use those temporal wrinkles and fill them with the things we love… then, when things got intense, bad, or routine, we could simply slip through the fabric of Time and stay as long as we wished, refreshing ourselves on the positive things.[4]

I have had positive response to the song. When I start to sing, I often get smiles or shocked expressions from patients who seem to feel the incongruity of having a man in a lab coat with a clown nose singing to them in the hospital. But then, they start to listen to what the song is saying. Listening, they start to get silent and thoughtful, as Stephanie does today. A change in expression indicates they have begun to suspect there is method in my madness and a message for them in the song.

Not surprisingly, it is Bob Zentz' intention that his songs provoke thoughtful reflection on the meaning of life. As he says in the liner notes,

> A song is a mirror of the Universe in which we exist, reflecting the history of the past and the possibilities of the future. To sing the past and dream the future unifies us with the Outer Spaces of eternal intelligence and universal existence. To be one with yourself is to be one with the Universe.[5]

In singing his song, I borrow his intention to provoke reflection. And when, for a moment, a patient gets a dreamy, far off look as I am singing, I figure she has been charmed by the magic of the song and has dived into the intimate depths of the soul or vaulted into the immensity of Outer Space, where in either place the line of time bends back on itself. It seems if there are others in the room, they, too, go somewhere in their minds. Sometimes when I am singing, parents close their eyes and nod their heads in identification with the wish for a private place of respite. Sometimes they shed a tear that shows me they are deeply moved by the wish of the song or possibly, by the wish they hold that their child might find such a place of internal strength.

Dr. Merryandrew: And that's what you've got, a wrinkle in time, a light shield, a place where you can go inside and get rested and strong. Go back out, you're on the highway… Where'd you put that key I gave you?… Good. What are you going to do with it? Where are you going to keep it?... In your pocket!?! … Does your mother ever wash your clothes? One day you're going to forget the key in your pocket. She washes your pants and out it goes in the wash… I'll tell you what to do with it. Put it on a chain around your neck. No one will see it. But when you need it, you'll have it… I'll tell you a secret. There are thousands of people walking around Greensboro with keys to the Shield of Light around their necks. You're a society of people with keys to the Shield of Light around your necks. You can find each other, join together, form a movement, change the world. We need people with keys to the Shield of Light to change the world.

This is the most generically diverse experience I offer patients. It jumps around from clowning to mime to explanations of time and slack rope walking to song to advice and even to a call to action – a meandering rhythm of diversion, a highwire act of incongruities. I try to keep it moving and have the focus shift before the patient's interest slacks. As the focus shifts, the mood changes between humor and seriousness, purposefulness and mockery. Considering its diversity, it still seems remarkable to me that this was the first routine that evolved out of my experience with patients and as it came together, that it seemed to have a quality Marcel Marceau, one of my mentors in performance, liked to call "light-heaviness."

The instance in which I heard Marceau use this term, light-heaviness, was when he was critiquing a performance I had just done for him in the context of a professional seminar of mimes from around the country who had come to learn from his mastery. The performance piece was simply titled, "Esau." It was a movement portrayal of Esau hunting for game to offer his father, Isaac, in exchange for his blessing. It also expressed Esau's despair at learning that his blessing was stolen by his brother, Jacob. Marceau himself performed a well-known piece based on the story of Cain and Abel, so I thought he might appreciate my translation into mime of the story of Jacob and Esau. He was generous with me this day, did not challenge any part of the piece, and told the whole seminar there was nothing much to say when the performance was entirely successful. But then, since he was loquacious when not on the mime stage, Marceau did go on to say what was important to the performance was its quality of "light-heaviness." He explained that when you want to express something of great seriousness onstage, it is important to bring grace and lightness to the performance, so that it does not become ponderous and burdensome for the audience. He made a point of recognizing that in performance, there is a principle of counterweight. He demonstrated that even when expressing an emotion like grief, which might ordinarily cause someone to fold over to hold the loss inside, it is important onstage to open up and give the emotion up and out so that the audience can read it.

So as my Shield of Light routine came together, I recognized I had learned the lesson well from Marceau so many years earlier. The piece takes the patient into some areas of seriousness, but moves back into humor before the mood can get ponderous.

When the kernel of the idea for the Shield of Light first came to me, I was looking to find representation for the sense of the importance of light to a sense of well-being. I have heard others say that when looking at someone they can detect the person's aura, which is a color radiance around a person. But I do not see auras and make no claim one way or the other that the Shield of Light has to do with aura reading and that kind of clairvoyance. My sense of the light around the body is simpler than that. To give it verbal expression, I would say I find there is a radiance around someone who has a strong sense of well-being. We say of some people with that radiance that "she lights up the room." When I had the idea for this piece, I was hoping to help patients imagine themselves into the radiance of well-being. I wanted patients to feel enveloped by light and that the light that enveloped them was a protective shield. Initially I did not say anything about thousands of people walking around the city with keys to the Shield of Light around their necks. But as I gave out more and more keys to patients and I began to realize that there were a lot of patients walking around our city with keys I had given them, I began to imagine for myself a gathering of those with the radiance of well-being. The image started to promise transformation on a societal scale to match the transformation I imagined for individual patients. But I did not want to make a whole case for that; just drop it in at the end to give the Shield of Light a meaningful twist beyond the personal.

Stephanie and her mother have taken it all in lightly today. Stephanie seemed amused by it all, growing quiet during the song, but good-naturedly playing along at the end when I told her to put the key on a chain around her neck by making the gestures of doing that.

If a patient is still in the hospital the next day, I may ask her if she still has the key around her neck. But I seldom know whether patients remember that they have a key to the Shield of Light after they leave the hospital.

Whether the patient responds with amusement or with reflective seriousness and whether or not the patient carries the memory of the Shield of Light into daily life is not my concern. Either way I know I have given her a key to the Shield of Light and she has received it. Maybe in a difficult moment of life the recollection of the Shield of Light will stir a feeling for what can sustain.

Chapter Four

The Golden Feather

The Pediatric unit is on the sixth floor, which is the top floor, of the older section of the hospital. One year during my nine years here, a large red-tailed hawk made frequent visits to the window ledges outside the rooms and to the rooftop of a lower section of the building just below our windows. Gazing out of a window at the hawk on the window ledge or with its wings spread wide to absorb vitamin D from the sun on the rooftop below, one had the sensation of venturing into or maybe invading the hawks habitat. I always felt privileged when I caught a glimpse of this majestic feathered presence of power and wildness. And I was not alone in feeling that way.

One day the hawk landed on the window ledge of the room outside of which we are now standing. When I entered the room, the patient was sitting on the couch which is built into the niche below the window. Framed in the window, the bird was inches from the patient's face. As if he were behind mirrored glass, he seemed unaware that he was being observed at close range. I knew better than to interrupt the child's rapture at the visit of this wild creature to his room. I watched with the child in the stillness and silence that overcomes me when I am outside among wild beings. And I figured the well-being of the patient was best served by the humbling grandeur of wild nature.

Unfortunately, I have not seen the hawk lately and do not expect to see him when we enter this room. I will have to see how to serve the patient without that help from the outside.

The boy in this room is twelve years old. For a change, instead of mom, his dad is sitting with him when I enter the room. After I introduce myself in the usual way, I do not get much of a feeling for what to do. He seems taciturn and withdrawn and his dad is just watching me silently as if he does not know what to make of me. But neither of them is asking me to leave, so I take a minute to get more of a reading of him by asking how he is doing. He tells me he is feeling bored. This is not uncommon for a boy of twelve who finds himself stuck in a hospital bed for a few days. Sometimes for help understanding what to do for them, I ask patients who are bored what they might rather be doing than sitting in the hospital. But this time, I decide to try to get a rise out of him with a little self-mockery.

Dr. Merryandrew: What? You don't find doctors and nurses and clowns like me coming and going in your room exciting and a welcome change from your everyday life?

That gets a wry smile; after all he is twelve years old and entitled to regard an old man like me as rather lame. I jump into the opening.

Dr. Merryandrew: How 'bout I tell you a story? Do you like stories? (He gives a wishy-washy nod.) I'll tell you a story about a hunter. Have you ever been hunting?
Matthew: (Smiling) Yeah.
Matthew's Dad: Matthew, tell him about the eight-point buck you got the first time you went out.

Since we get patients from around our region, which includes rural farms and forests just outside the city, it is not unusual to hear that a young boy is already learning to hunt with his father. Although I am not a hunter, I have heard several different stories about hunting excursions. More often than not they are like play-by-play stories of baseball games because the tellers have not yet found a way to communicate the tension and excitement and, in hunting, the ambivalence they may have felt. After listening to Matthew's story of his first hunting trip and the huge buck, I begin my own story.

Dr. Merryandrew: My story about a hunter is a little different than yours. But before I tell you the story of the hunter, I have to tell you all my stories are old stories. All my stories are old stories, not because they were told long ago or because they are about things that happened long ago. They are old stories because I learned from the old masters. The old masters knew that life is full of magic and miracle, that sometimes people can turn into animals and sometimes animals can turn into people. They knew that animals and people could communicate with each other, or as we say, they could talk. Maybe you have heard some of those old stories where straw or nettles are spun into gold. Maybe if we listen to the old stories, we will know what the old masters knew. Maybe if more people hear the old stories, there will be more people around who know that life is full of magic and miracle.

I did not introduce my storytelling like this until I had been telling stories to patients for awhile. From the start of my work in the hospital, however,

I knew that storytelling would be a part of what I offered patients. "I am the doctor who treats your ills with tales and folly." Stories, I thought, everyone likes a good story. We can be entertained or escape into an engaging story. And stories do so much of the work of psychic life. Story is the way we bring order to the chaotic experiences of living. Stories shape and reshape our identities. Stories give us a sense of meaning and purpose. They show us our good fortune and our fate. They weave us into our communities. How often we request, "Tell me a story" or "Tell me the story." We ask to hear bedtime stories as children and impart our wisdom in stories when we are old.

After I had some experience in the hospital, I recognized that storytelling was one of the best ways to engage young boys and teenagers who believed that they had outgrown childish things, which included clowns like me. But I also recognized that folktales and fairytales might receive the same disdain for the same reason. So I began to address that liability with an introduction that might subtly lift my tales from the context of the nursery into the realm of fantasy literature, which is a popular genre for young adults and adults in general. Also the introduction was a way, not so subtly, to say I am going to tell you a story, but a story is never just a story; it is a most important vehicle of meaning. And with academic credentials in the field of Folklore, my claim to have learned from the old masters was literally true.

Dr. Merryandrew: This is a story about a hunter. He was riding through a forest on a horse of power. Do you know about the horses of power?... On the steppes of Asia, which is a big land mass stretching 5,000 miles from Hungary and Romania in the West to Mongolia and Manchuria in the East, there were herds of horses. You probably know there were no horses on this continent before the Spanish brought them to America. But on the steppes of Asia there were great herds of horses. These herds were led by great stallions. The stallions fought with each other and only the strongest and smartest survived. These stallions were so smart that they could outwit the greatest strategists of the world. Do you know who they are? Not human beings. The greatest strategists of the world are the wolves. Wolves taught human beings the strategies of war. Wolves travel in packs. When they are hunting, the pack surrounds their prey; they send out decoys to distract their target before they close in for the kill. But these great stallions could outwit the wolves and lead their herds to safety. They say they were so smart that they could communicate with human beings; or as we say, they could talk.

In my earlier performance career and as a teacher, I had developed a repertoire of favorite stories that I liked to tell. I tried telling several of the stories I already knew in the new setting of the hospital, but I lighted on this one as an early favorite in my hospital repertoire and I started to expand and embellish it as I told and retold it. As the telling evolved, historical and geographical accuracy was not my concern. Nor did I feel I had to adhere precisely to the structure of the tale or the style in which I initially encountered it. I learned a version of this Russian tale when, many years ago, I was reading a book by Michael Meade called *Men and the Water of Life: Initiation and the Tempering of Men.* The text had nothing about the origin of the horse of power. But I decided to give the horse of power more attention both for the sake of the story and the patient. Since I experience the natural world as healing, anything I can do to inspire a richer connection with nature for the patient seems beneficial to me. So I like to spend a little time empowering the horse of power.

Dr. Merryandrew: The hunter was riding on one of those great stallions, a horse of power. He was riding through a forest. He had been in this forest many times before. As usual, he saw squirrels running up and down the trunks of trees, raccoons in the branches, rabbits and foxes hopping behind the bushes. But then he realized there were no birds. He had always seen birds in the forest before. But this day, he listened and heard no birds singing. Where were all the birds? Then he rode around a curve in the trail he was on and there on the ground was a golden feather.

Then he knew what had happened. The firebird had come into the forest, the great magical mystical bird. When the firebird enters the forest, all the other birds leave. He looked at the feather on the ground and thought to himself, "No one has ever found a feather from the firebird. If I pick up that feather and bring it to the king, the king will reward me with gold and silver." In these old stories, you have to understand, a king is not, as we might think, necessarily someone at the head of a monarchy. As in this story, when the story calls someone a king, it means the person is someone of power and wealth and influence. That's what the hunter meant when he said to himself, "The king will reward me."

So the hunter rode up to the feather, got down off his horse and went to pick up the feather. Just as he was about to pick it up, the horse said to him, "Do not pick up that feather. If you pick up that feather, you will know fear and trouble." But the hunter did not listen to him. He picked up the feather, put it in his hat, got back on his horse, and rode to the palace of the king. He carried it down the great hall to the throne room and gave it to the king.

The king took the feather. " Ah, a feather from the firebird. This is truly a great gift for a king. No other king has a feather from the firebird." The hunter knelt down the way you do before a king to receive his reward. But the king did not reward him. Instead he said, "If you can find a feather from the firebird, surely you can capture the bird itself and bring it back to me... alive. If you do not, my sword will sing through the air and sever your head from your shoulders."

The hunter went out of the throne room down the great hall to his horse in tears. How could he capture the firebird? No one had ever even found a feather from the firebird. It was impossible to capture the bird. When the horse saw him, he said,

"I told you if you picked up that feather, you would know fear and trouble... But your trouble is not yet. Go back to the king and ask the king for three lengths of rope and for a hundred sacks of grain to be spread in the field outside the palace tomorrow morning."

The next morning, the hunter was up in a tree in the field outside the palace, hidden by the leaves. All around the tree the hundred sacks of grain were opened and spread on the ground. The horse was slowly grazing in the field. All of a sudden, the leaves on the tree began to blow and the branches swayed. The leaves flipped upside down and showed their silvery undersides the way they do in a storm. Then out of the forest came the firebird, the magical mystical bird, and lighted in the field and began to peck at the grain. The horse kept grazing slowly in the field, all the time moving closer to the bird. Then all of a sudden it put its hoof down on the birds wing and held it down. The hunter came down from the tree with the three lengths of rope, threw the rope around the bird, bound it tight, and threw the bird on his back.

It was a big bird, but as we all know, birds have hollow bones so they can fly. So the bird was not heavy. The hunter got back on his horse, rode to the palace and carried the firebird down the great hall to the throne room, where the king opened a great cage in the throne room and locked the bird inside, alive.

"Ah, my friend, you have done well. You have captured the firebird. This is truly a great gift for a king," said the king. The hunter waited for his reward… But the king did not reward him. Instead he said, "If you can capture the firebird, it will not be difficult for you to go across the world to where the red sun rises out of the blue sea and bring back the beautiful Princess Vassilisa to be my bride. And if you do not, my sword will sing through the air and sever your head from your shoulders."

The hunter heard this and feared for his life. It was said that the Princess Vassilisa was the daughter of a wizard. Her father had put an enchantment on her. Many men had gone across the world to win her hand in marriage. None had returned. Again the hunter went out of the throne room, down the great hall to his horse in tears. When the horse saw him, he said, "I told you if you picked up that feather, you would know fear and trouble… But your trouble is not yet. Go back to the king and ask the king for a tent and for a sack of food and a sack of drink. And tomorrow morning we will go across the world and see what we can do." In those days, food and wine were carried in sacks made of animal skins. The wine sack was an animal bladder.

The next morning, rolled and strapped to the back of the saddle was a great tent. Down one side of the saddle in a saddle bag was a sack of food. Down the other side of the saddle in a saddle bag was a sack of drink. Off they went like lightning with flames sparking from the horse's hooves before them and flames sparking from the horse's hooves behind them.

Over hill and vale
On ancient trails
Through windswept meadows
Rain misted mountains
Through haunted forests

Shining streams
Past the cave of ghosts
And the horn and ivory gates of dreams

Till they came to the other side of the world where the red sun rises out of the blue sea. They went down to the beach. Out on the sea in a silver boat with golden oars sat a beautiful princess.

The hunter set up the tent on the beach. It was a beautiful tent with silver sides and a golden roof and all around the sides of the tent were illustrated the stories of old. In those days, a great tent was a sign of wealth and power. And anyone could see this was the tent of a king. The hunter laid out a blanket on the beach in front of the tent. He set the food and drink that he had brought with him on the blanket. It was a wonderful feast. Then he sat down on the blanket and waited.

Soon the princess in the silver boat with the golden oars rowed the boat into the beach, drew it up on the beach, got out and came and sat down with the hunter on the blanket. Together they feasted on the food and drink that the hunter had brought with him. They talked and laughed as they feasted. They enjoyed the afternoon together. As you might guess, the princess was very beautiful and charming. And the hunter was happy to be sitting with her by the sea and forgot why he had traveled across the world.

Now as they were enjoying the afternoon, the Princess Vassilisa looked over at the tent and asked about what was pictured all around the sides. The hunter answered, "They are illustrations of the old stories told by the old masters in my kingdom. All the stories the old masters told were full of magic and miracle."

He told her one of those stories. When he had finished, she asked to hear another... and after that one, another. When the hunter finished the third tale, she said, "I feel I have entered a forest of dreams and wonders. These are the stories of your kingdom? Can you bring me there? I would like to visit this land of magic and miracle."

"Then I will bring you there," he answered.

The hunter gathered up the remains of the feast and put them back in the saddle bags. He rolled the blanket and the tent and tied both to the saddle. He lifted the princess onto the saddle with him. Then off they went like lightning with flames sparking from the horse's hooves before them and flames sparking from the horse's hooves behind them.

Over hill and vale
On ancient trails
Through windswept meadows
Rain misted mountains
Through haunted forests

Shining streams
Past the cave of ghosts
And the horn and ivory gates of dreams

Till they came to the palace. The hunter got down and lifted the princess off the horse.

"This is the palace of our kingdom," the hunter told the princess.

He led the princess down the great hall into the throne room. The king was very pleased to see them and spoke immediately of his pleasure. "My friend, you have done what I asked. You have brought the Princess Vassilisa to be my bride. I am greatly pleased," he said. He reached into his chest of gold and silver and brought out a sack of gold and a sack of silver to reward the hunter. But just as he was about to give the hunter the sack of gold, the princess interrupted.

"What is happening?" asked the princess. She looked at the hunter in disbelief. The hunter looked back at her uneasily as if he wished to offer explanation, but just nodded his head and kept silent.

The king spoke. "You are here in my kingdom. I have had you brought from your world to mine to be my bride. You will be my queen. We will rule the kingdom together."

"No," said the princess, still staring at the hunter. "I cannot marry anyone unless I have my own wedding

dress which is hidden in a chest under a rock at the bottom of my sea. My father has put an enchantment on me. If I marry anyone without my own wedding dress, the one I marry will die."

The king heard this and put the gold and the silver back in the chest. He said to the hunter, "My friend, you must go back across the world to where the red sun rises out of the blue sea and bring back this chest with the wedding dress. And if you do not…" You know what he said; he threatened him with death.

Again the hunter went out of the throne room down the great hall to his horse, fearing for his life. When the horse saw him, he said, "I told you if you picked up that feather, you would know fear and trouble… But your trouble is not yet. Tomorrow morning we will go across the world and see what we can do."

The next morning, off they went like lightning with flames sparking from the horse's hooves before them and flames sparking from the horse's hooves behind them.

> *Over hill and vale*
> *On ancient trails*
> *Through windswept meadows*
> *Rain misted mountains*
> *Through haunted forests*
> *Shining streams*

Past the cave of ghosts
And the horn and ivory gates of dreams

Till they came to the other side of the world where the red sun rises out of the blue sea. They went down to the beach, the very same beach where the hunter had set up the tent before. There on the beach, crawling on the beach, was a crab. The horse went right up to the crab and put its hoof on the crab's back and held it down.

"Do not give me death," the crab called out.

"I will not," the horse said, "if you do this task for me. Go down to the bottom of the sea and bring back the chest that is hidden under a rock at the bottom of the sea."

This was the King of Crabs. He called out to all the other crabs, lobsters and starfish in the sea. They came out of the sea onto the beach. The beach was teeming with crabs, lobsters and starfish. The King of Crabs told them what they must do. Then they went back into the sea. For a moment by the shore it looked like the water was boiling; there was so much activity in the surf... Then it became calm and quiet... Then suddenly out of the sea, like a small volcano, the chest rose and broke the waves and slowly moved toward the beach. When it reached the beach, the hunter picked it up, got back on his horse, and off they went like lightning with flames sparking from the horse's hooves before them and flames sparking from the horse's hooves behind them.

> *Over hill and vale*
> *On ancient trails*
> *Through windswept meadows*
> *Rain misted mountains*
> *Through haunted forests*
> *Shining streams*
> *Past the cave of ghosts*
> *And the horn and ivory gates of dreams*

When they came to the palace, the hunter got down from his horse with the chest and carried the chest down the great hall. As he carried it down the great hall, the hunter pictured in his mind the afternoon by the sea when he and the princess had talked and laughed together. He stopped in the great hall as if he were dreaming. When he almost dropped the chest, he remembered where he was and his fear of the king's sword. He brought the chest into the throne room and set it down right before the princess and as he did, he looked directly into her eyes. She met his gaze and for a moment, he saw delight flicker in her eyes as she looked directly into his. Then the hunter turned away from her to face the king. He knelt down to receive his reward.

The king spoke. "Ah, my friend, you have done well. You have done everything I asked." He reached into his chest of gold and silver, and brought out two sacks of gold and two sacks of silver. The hunter waited to receive his reward at last, though now he felt no gold or silver was as valuable as the light in the princess' eyes.

Just as the king was about to hand the hunter the first sack of gold, the princess spoke, "No, the one who brought me to this world must be put to death." The hunter could not believe what he heard. He turned to look at the princess; with his eyes he asked her, "What is happening?" But her eyes looked back coldly into his as if she had not read the question in his own. And he wondered how her eyes could go so quickly from the softness of delight to hard and cold.

The king put the sacks of gold and silver back in his chest. He ordered guards to hold the hunter. He sentenced the hunter to be put to death in a vat of boiling oil in a public execution in the morning before the wedding the next day. The hunter heard his sentence. He begged the king, "Please let me say goodbye to my horse." The king allowed it. With the guards at his side, the hunter went out of the throne room down the great hall to his horse.

He said to his horse, "Goodbye, my dear friend, we will no longer ride through the green fields, over the high mountains, through the dark forests and the *shining streams. Tomorrow I will be put to death in a vat of boiling oil in a public execution in the morning."*

The horse looked at him and said, "I told you if you picked up that feather, you would know fear and trouble... ... ... But your trouble is not yet. When the guards bring you to the vat of boiling oil, break away from them and run and jump into the vat of boiling oil yourself."

Strange advice, don't you think? Would you take it?...
Matthew: (nonplused to be asked this question) I'm not sure.

Dr. Merryandrew: (To Matthew's dad): What about you?

Matthew's Dad: I guess I would take the advice. The horse seems to have been helpful so far.

Dr. Merryandrew: I don't know if I would; I don't even like taking a hot shower. But the hunter had no choice.

The next morning the guards brought the hunter to the courtyard of the palace. All around the courtyard were arrayed all the people of the kingdom. There were men and women there. They were nobles and peasants, farmers and shepherds and hunters, wheelwrights, blacksmiths, potters, tavern keepers and inn keepers, cooks and bakers, cobblers and carpenters, poets and apothecaries. The king and the princess were there too. In the center of the courtyard, there was a vat of oil boiling over a blazing fire.

The hunter broke away from the guards, ran and dived into the vat of boiling oil. He went down into the oil. He bobbed up, but went down again, like a drowning man… But then, he bobbed up again. Not only did he bob up; he leapt out of the vat. And he was standing beside the vat… alive… Not only was he alive; he was more handsome than he had been when he dived into the vat. There was a golden light around him. All the people saw it. You could hear the whole assembled crowd gasp at once, Ahhh. The king and Vassilisa saw it.

The king thought to himself, "This must be magic oil. I too would like to become a golden being." So the king ran and dived into the vat of boiling oil. He went down once and bobbed up and went down a second time, like a drowning man… But then he too bobbed up a second time and leapt out of the vat… But the king… was turned into a great bear that circled once around the courtyard and ran off into the forest and was never seen again.

The wedding had been scheduled for 12 noon, but there was no king to marry the princess. It was decided in that moment by all the people of the kingdom who were there in the courtyard that the hunter should marry the princess and he should become their king. So it happened. The hunter and Vassilisa were married. At the wedding everyone in the kingdom could see that the hunter and the princess were happy to be in each other's arms as they danced. And this time the hunter was sure he understood the flicker of delight in the princess' eyes.

Together the hunter and the princess went on to rule the kingdom as king and queen for many years. They were great and generous rulers.

Now, what do think their first task as king and queen was after their wedding?...

Matthew: Maybe they went after the bear.

Dr. Merryandrew: No, I already mentioned the bear was never seen again.

Matthew's Dad: (Silently shakes his head to indicate he cannot imagine what the king and queen did.)

Dr. Merryandrew: I'll tell you. They went back to the throne room, opened the great cage and let the firebird, the magical mystical bird, fly free. As far as I know, it is still flying in a forest somewhere in the world.

The hunter ruled a long time. When he died, they buried him in the ground with his horse of power. They say many hunters of old are buried in the ground with their horses of power where they are waiting for a time when the world needs them. Then they are going to come riding out of the ground to save the world... If you ask me, that time is coming soon.

There's a story for you. You know, the great thing about these old stories is you can place yourself in them at different stages of your life. That way they give you a sense of where you are in the story of your life. Are you riding across the world to bring back a beautiful princess? Are you trying to recover a hidden chest with something important inside in a far off part of the world? Are you expecting a reward for something you have accomplished? Are you hoping to capture a magical mystical being? Are you in a vat of boiling oil, wondering whether you are going to be turned into a golden being or a bear? Are you about to pick up a golden feather when you have been warned not to? Where are you right now in the story?

Matthew does not answer my rhetorical question, but he looks as if he is thinking about it. We can leave him thinking.

I am sure different metaphorical interpretations might help to explain the impact of this story on listeners. I believe Michael Meade offered an interpretation of that kind in the chapter of the book in which I first encountered his variant of the tale. However, I do not remember his interpretation. Besides it would likely seem irrelevant to the transformed tale that I have crafted from the tale to which I was introduced. As a storyteller, I am not inclined toward interpretation. It seems too academic to me as a storyteller to think analytically and critically about a story. I also do not want to inhibit my freedom and enthusiasm in the telling of the tale. Moreover, I feel interpretation would displace my effort to account for the immediacy of the encounter with the patient. So neither patients nor I have ever entered into interpretations in our exchange. I only go so far in that direction as carried in the words of the introduction and the rhetorical questions asked at the end. It seems to me to be enough to recognize that in times of uncertainty and crisis engendered by disease, stories serve to weave patients into a sense of their place in the tapestry of life, meaning, relation and belonging.

In telling a story, I experience the telling as a dramatic action shared between the patient and me. Something of significance takes place between us. And a relation is established. The story creates a sort of bond through the shared imagination similar to the tensile connection between a patient and me in the Shield of Light. This particular story of "The Golden Feather" actually has storytelling serve as just such an act of relation between the hunter and the princess. The hunter tells the Princess Vassilisa some of the old stories illustrated on the sides of the tent. In telling those stories, he establishes a relation between himself and the princess, a relation of trust, and he wins her over to accompanying him back across the world to his kingdom. Something happens as a result of the storytelling. Similarly telling a story to a patient in the hospital is an act of relation between myself and the patient.

The relation between myself and the patient has a certain degree of intimacy. When I tell a story to a large group, inevitably the telling has a more presentational style. By contrast, in the intimate setting of a one-to-one exchange, the storytelling has more of the feel of conversation. I may even stop to check with the patient about his needs in the moment – pain level, need to sleep or take a bathroom break, or to call a nurse to attend to an IV.

The most common experience I can compare to telling a story at the bedside of a patient in the hospital is telling or reading a bedtime story to a child. In our own family sometimes we read a favorite picture book at bedtime to our children, sometimes we told stories that my wife or I made up ourselves or stories from our own lives. As many parents know, a bedtime story is a good way to settle children at the end of an active day and to ease the transition into sleep. A story becomes an intimate exchange and the bedtime hour is enveloped in the soothing experience of shared imagination.

In my own childhood, my father often spun stories around a single trickster character whose long comical name began with Okeechokee. The sound of the name alone, which my father often strung out with a number of epithets, would thrill me with a mix of humor and mystery even before the story began. To the child I was then the content of the stories, was never as important as the pleasure my father and I took in the shared imagination. I remember my father laughing at times as he discovered a turn in the narrative he was creating and I shared his glee.

I picked up the tradition of telling stories to my children. My daughter, Liz, and I still share a memory of a story I spun out over many nights about a little girl who was a doll maker and her father. I remember the story having a Dickensian feeling to it, but night after night, as I strung it out, neither of us knew where it was going. It did not matter because we were inside the adventure of the story together and were mutually delighted to be sharing that adventure together. Then something interrupted the rhythm of the evenings in the sequence of the nights during which the story was evolving and it never was completed. And yet it had already served so well for us that those nights remain an important memory for both my daughter and me. It remains in our memories as a significant experience of our close relation.

A story told at the bedside of a patient is likewise a significant experience shared. A verbal event has taken place for the two of us in the space between us and has shaped the hour into a relation. The impact of the intimacy is what matters first even before the impact of the narrative sinks in. Just to have shared the imagination of a story seems to affirm something fundamental to the human search for meaning.

When I tell a patient afterwards, he can find himself in the story, I am not just reinforcing memory of the episodes of the story. I am not implying that life will follow the trajectory of the tale I have told. I am emphasizing, that in the drift of our days there is meaning, even in the drift of these days, maybe especially in the drift of these days in the hospital, there is meaning. No day, no moment need ever be lost. To see one's reflection in a story is to catch a glimpse of who one is and in that glimpse, to catch a flicker of meaning in one's life. You can see yourself in the story because your life is a wondrous story.

Chapter Five

Jamie I: Love Is Something If You Give It Away

As my work in the hospital evolved, I felt I needed a bridge between Dr. Merryandrew and younger patients. Children eight or nine years old and up could engage with me in long routines like the Shield of Light or long stories like "The Golden Feather," but I found I needed a different way of connecting with the younger ones. It seemed like a good opportunity to introduce puppetry into my hospital repertoire. I was hopeful I could get help with the young ones by eliciting the help of a puppet friend. I figured that a diminutive partner could facilitate relationship with diminutive patients.

Since I work alone, I was enthusiastic about finding a partner with whom to share the challenges of attending to patients, even if that partner was a puppet. Over the years, I worked with puppets in other circumstances — stuffed animals, hand puppets and marionettes – partners in performance. The children's show entitled, "Stick to Your Dreams," that I toured for many years, always began with a sequence with a Steiff toy monkey. I also made my own puppets for a full length show that I created with funding from the NEA. And as a mask maker and mask performer, I know the magic of animating the inanimate.

Influences between mask and performer or puppet and performer magically flow both ways. Whenever I perform in a mask or with a puppet, I experience that neither mask nor puppet will be manipulated as an inert object. Each one has its own interiority and makes its own demands. If, as a performer, I ever try to dominate a mask or puppet as a wholly lifeless object, the mask or puppet saps my energy. I feel it is my own body that has become inanimate. I have learned that the unique life of a mask or a puppet needs to be honored. Performing with a mask or puppet is a dynamic interchange with a very vital entity. So I was excited about the thought of having a puppet as a dynamic intermediary between the children and me because I knew that if I brought a puppet into patients' rooms, I would be entering with an animated partner. Of course I had to consider who I wanted to invite to be my partner.

I auditioned several candidates. That is, I tried out several different puppets with patients. I tried animal hand puppets: a bald eagle, a bat, a monkey and a green turtle whose neck contracts to pull its head inside its shell. But I rejected all the hand puppets because I felt that hand puppets wanted more aesthetic distance to come alive and I needed a companion I could bring right up to the bedside. At close range, I felt my hand puppets seemed too attached to me, not independent enough. Marionettes had more promise. All my marionettes are human characters: an old clown, Little Red Riding Hood, and a few young clowns. I expected to select the old clown dressed in black checked pants, a yellow vest with red buttons, a red and white striped bowtie, a black tailcoat, white gloves, and black dancing shoes. He has carrot orange hair and the colorful makeup of an August clown – whiteface, painted red nose, lips and cheeks, splashes of blue on chin and forehead, and additional highlights of yellow. His features are sculpted and pronounced – pointed chin, well-shaped mouth, high cheekbones, wide eyes with heavy lids, high arching eyebrows, and a prominent well-articulated nose. His appearance delivers a strong impact. He is a dapper gent and seems genial enough to be a suitable foil and partner for me. But I was surprised to discover after days of auditions one of the young clowns was to be my partner.

The young one seemed to win the hearts of children immediately because he himself has a very child-like appearance. He is very simply made. He wears red overalls with two large pockets. Clipped to the outside of the left pocket with a yellow clothes pin he carries a white rag decorated with colorful polka dots. He also sports a small yellow banana-shaped bead where the right strap for his overalls might be buttoned. His shirt has horizontal blue and white stripes and billows like his overalls. He has a green bowtie attached to the top of his shirt. On his head, he wears a wide-brimmed felt hat with a red string band around it and a yellow flower in the band on the right side. His straw-colored hair sticks out under the hat. His hands are fashioned from dowels that have been rounded. His shoes, likewise, are plain wood without paint. They are rectangular in shape, rounded at the four corners, domed on the top side, and flat on the bottom. His pants hold his feet on by gathering around dowels stuck into the tops of his shoes. His face is shaped from a simple rounded wooden egg of the same wood as his hands and shoes. On it are painted two black dots for eyes with small black lines above for eyebrows. The red line of his lips is outlined with a broad sweep of white which gives him an open smile. In the center of his face his nose is a bulbous red knob. The simple elements of his appearance give him the appeal of innocence and make him immediately endearing . He is a towering twelve inches tall and speaks and sings in a falsetto voice.

But before I account for how he became a dominant figure in the room and an equal in our partnership, I need to add a note about what I brought to the experience of partnering with a puppet.

For several years my younger daughter and I would spend time creating worlds with her dolls. A favorite activity was to pretend all the dolls were in a class at school. We set them in doll desks we had or in front of block tables and gave them daily assignments. Then we would help them complete their assignments in small folios made from writing paper. Sometimes too, the dolls would make meals at the play stove, play games or just play freely in an imagined world. One time we tied ribbons to a pole and had all the dolls holding a ribbon in a circle around the pole for a May Day celebration. Whatever filled the afternoon was always very engaging play, so engaging that one time at the beginning of the afternoon, my daughter picked out one doll from the rest and set her in the middle of the room. Then we sat back and waited to see what this lone doll would decide to do. We just sat there watching and waiting in anticipation. Of course nothing happened. But we still sat there waiting, until finally we burst into laughter. The laughter was a laughter of delight. We were not at all embarrassed by our foolish expectation. Somewhere inside it, our laughter said to us both, "Isn't it wonderful that our imaginations bring so much life into the afternoons." But there was more than that in the laughter. Although we recognized in the moment of laughter that we breathed life in the doll, we also knew that she had her own personality. That is why we selected her. Some part of our laughter acknowledged that we were anticipating that specific doll's contribution to our afternoon, not the contributions of any others. Years later, my daughter, Liz, and I can still evoke that joyful laughter by remembering, "Remember the time we watched one doll do nothing?"

When I came to the hospital, I brought with me those memories of shared afternoons with my daughter and the lesson they taught me. For a child engaged in play no object is ever inanimate. I arrived at the hospital aware that any object brought into imaginative exchange is alive and has an interiority of its own. No ritual transubstantiation needed. And maybe as in tribal societies around the world where puppets are used by shamans, a puppet could bring a bit of healing power into a hospital room, as well.

But I had a lot to learn about the power of puppetry. The first thing I learned is that a puppet has his own mind and speaks for himself. One morning when he had just begun to come with me, my marionette asked a patient her name. She answered and in turn asked him his name. "My name is Jamie," he blurted out, startling me with his quick reply. Later on, I rationalized the origin of the name for myself. Jaime (of course, pronounced differently than Jamie) was the name of a patient I saw early on in my work who had been enormously helpful in teaching me how to serve patients. Jamie was also the name of the child hero in my favorite book of my childhood. Later I also added a further rationale to these. Jamie has the same name as a doctor in the Pediatric Emergency Department, whom I admire as a physician and as a person, who fortunately, does not mind sharing her name with my puppet. But I dare say, it was really Jamie who named himself.

Eventually I started introducing Jamie as my son and he started introducing me as his dad. This was felicitous in ways I could not have anticipated. For one, it gave him an available background story when asked questions about his family, such as, where were his mother and siblings and what kind of a dog does he have. Like anyone with a mischievous dog, he has been able to tell stories about what his dog does. And he is happy to elicit stories about other people's dogs.

The father-son relationship between us also contributed to Jamie's reflections on his own reality and what defines a person's identity.

Jamie: Hi, who are you?

Natasha (patient): I'm Natasha. Who are you?

Jamie: That's a really nice name, Natasha. Can I have your name? My name is Jamie. This guy over here in the white coat is my dad, Dr. Merryandrew? I'll tell you what, we'll exchange names. I'll take yours and you'll take mine.

Natasha: That's silly. Besides, Natasha is a girl's name and you are a boy.

Jamie: It doesn't matter. There's a doctor around here named Jamie, the same as me, and she's a girl.

Natasha: That's different. Jamie can be either. Anyway, I'm keeping my name. You can't have it.

Jamie: Well, OK. How are you feeling, Natasha?

Natasha: I'm good.

Jamie: If you're good, why are you here? Do you know this is a hospital? People come here when they're not feeling good. Maybe I oughta send you home.
Natasha: You can't do that. You're just a puppet.
Jamie: What do you mean, I'm just a puppet? I'm a real boy and I could tell your nurse to send you home.
Natasha: No, you can't. You're not real. You're just a toy.

Natasha is five years old. Like some young children her age, her world is defined literally. Things are as they are named. Accordingly, a puppet by definition is not allowed to have a dynamic life of his own. Or so she has been led to believe according to the rules she is beginning to learn about order in her world. But that order is not so formed in her for as a child her world is still animated. She has not really crossed from the enchanted world of childhood into the rational world of adulthood. The irony of the exchange is that she is arguing with a puppet and asserting that he is not real. Against what she argues, she has become engaged in an exchange with him that is not unlike a child's characteristic exchange with another child. Despite her recently learned categories of what is real and what is not, she has been drawn into relationship. She insistently tells Jamie he is not real while engaging him in a conversation as if he is very real indeed.

Jamie: I am, too, real. Do you even know how you get to be real? The way you get to be real is if somebody loves you. And my dad loves me, so I'm real.

Jamie's explanation of how one gets to be real is borrowed from *The Velveteen Rabbit*, the classic children's book by Margery Williams Bianco.

Natasha: Well, I'm muscle and bone and you're wood.
Jamie: Muscle and bone doesn't make you real. And it certainly doesn't make you a real human being. Maybe you're a chicken. Are you a chicken?
Natasha: Of course I'm not a chicken. I don't have feathers or wings.
Jamie: Well, does anybody love you?
Natasha: Yes, somebody does. My momma and poppa love me. And my sister loves me. And my gramma and Pops love me. And my dog loves me.
Jamie: Ok then, I guess you're real same as me… Uh oh, who's this coming into the room? Oh, Hey Vickie. Are you here to give me a shot or to check vitals… Check vitals. Good. You can check my blood pressure first. Which arm do you want to check?

The day I was introduced around the Emergency Department by the director, it seemed that every nurse she introduced me to was named

"Vickie." By the fourth "Vickie" the director delivered the introduction with an apologetic shrug in acknowledgement of the repetition. When my orientation to the department was complete, I asked the director if all the nurses in the department were called "Vickie." She laughed and said it was just an accident of scheduling that day. But the experience of all those "Vickies," was the first suggestion I got that the Emergency Department had its own brand of absurd humor. Despite the traumas they sometimes confront, emergency nurses are upbeat and can be very funny. We had our droll storytellers and those who carried the burdens of the department with a light dose of irony. Occasionally one could hear a nurse tech kid one of the nurses, "Hey, Sam, how many lives did you save yesterday?" Not long after I started serving in the Emergency Department, I learned that the nurses kept a little notebook in which they recorded the outlandish diagnoses patients gave for coming to Emergency. In another notebook they made a list of the unusual names given to children who came through the doors to be seen. Readings from one of these notebooks were given in idle moments in the department. So it turned out, my encounter with the multiple "Vickies" was my early introduction to the myriad ways that the Emergency Department was not to be understood as a humorless place.

Vickie (Vickie responds to Jamie.): I don't think I have a cuff small enough for your arm, Jamie.
Jamie: Well, take my temperature, heart rate and oxygen then. I'm ready.
Vickie: I think I have to attend to Natasha, Jamie. She's the patient.
Jamie: Wait a second, Vickie. I need regular checkups when I'm working here. Are you telling me that I'm not important? That's not very nice.
Vickie: You're important, Jamie. But you're not the patient, Jamie, Natasha is… I can't believe I'm arguing with a puppet.
Jamie: Did you hear that, Natasha? Vickie thinks I'm a puppet. You better tell her I'm real. Tell Vickie how you get to be real.
Natasha: Jamie thinks he's real. He says if somebody loves you, you are real. He says his dad loves him, so he is real.
Jamie: See. I'm real. I'm not a puppet. Pinocchio is a puppet; I'm real… Aren't you real because someone loves you, Vickie?
Vickie: I don't know, Jamie.
Jamie: What do you mean, you don't know? This is

important. Didn't someone tell you they loved you?... Shucks, Vickie, we've got to see to this. We love you. My dad and I love you. Natasha loves you. Don't you, Natasha? So now you know you're real.

Vickie: Well, thanks, Jamie. I didn't know you had it in ya'… Now listen little man, step aside so I can take Natasha's vital signs. (Jamie and Dr. Merryandrew wait quietly while Vickie takes Natasha's vital signs, records them in the chart on the room computer and exits the room.)

Jamie: Well, Natasha, thank you for joining me and my dad in helping make sure Vickie knows she is real. We did our good deed for the day... Uh oh, now someone else is coming in to bother us. Who is this?

Dr. Jefferson: Hello, Natasha, I'm Dr. Jefferson. I'm the attending physician today. How are you feeling, Natasha?

Jamie: She's good. She told me she's good… Natasha, do you think this guy is a real doctor? He doesn't even have a white coat like my dad. How can he be a doctor?

Dr. Jefferson: Heh… heh… Hi, Jamie. Good to see you. Natasha didn't tell you she has a stomach ache?

Jamie: Nope, she didn't. Maybe just meeting me fixed it. Or maybe she gave it to me. Maybe you ought to check me, too.

Dr. Jefferson: (Dr. Jefferson puts his stethoscope near Jamie's stomach.) You're stomach sounds good, Jamie.

Now let me check Natasha.

Jamie: OK, Doctor… See you later, Natasha." (Jamie and Dr. Merryandrew exit the room. When Dr. Jefferson leaves the room, Jamie and Dr. Merryandrew return.)

Jamie: Natasha, do you think Dr. Jefferson is a real doctor?

Natasha: Of course he is; he's a good doctor.

Jamie: Good, I'm glad you like him… Who is that sitting in the chair against the wall next to your bed?

Natasha: That's Mom.

Jamie: There are so many people named Mom around here. It seems like it's a very popular name… Hi, I'm Jamie. This is my dad, Dr. Merryandrew.

Mom: Hi, Jamie. Hi, Doctor.

Jamie: Dr. Jefferson is really a good doctor. He'll get Natasha fixed up in no time. Don't worry.

Mom: He seems very nice.

Jamie: Well, before I leave you, can I sing you a song? Do you know "The Magic Penny?"

Natasha: No, how does it go?

Jamie: Love is something if you give it away,

>   *Give it away, give it away.*

>   *Love is something if you give it away,*

>   *You end up having more.*

>   *It's just like a magic penny,*

Hold it fast, you won't have any.
Lend it spend it and you'll have so many
They'll roll all over the floor.

Love is something if you give it away,
Give it away, give it away.
Love is something if you give it away,
You end up having more.

So let's go dancing till the break of day,
And if there's a piper, we can pay.
For love is something if you give it away,
You end up having more.

For love is something if you give it away,
Give it away, give it away.
Love is something if you give it away.
You end up having more.[6]

There's a song for you, Natasha.
Natasha: I liked it.
Mom: That's a nice song.
Jamie: Thank you. Be well, Natasha.

When he encounters a new patient for the first time in the Emergency Department, as he did today with Natasha, Jamie focuses on creating an atmosphere of sociability. As a garrulous convivial scamp, he tries to weave everyone in the room into interaction.

Anyone there or anyone who enters the room is fair game. His attitude is inclusive.

Sometimes Jamie can even leap a language barrier. For instance, one patient I saw each day after surgery spoke English very well, but his parents spoke almost no English. Sometimes the child would explain to the parents what was going on in our exchange. This seemed to be as much of a relationship as there could be with the family. But one day after meeting Jamie, the patient's father brought a simple dancing marionette with him when he came to visit. The marionette had come with the family from Mexico and wore a sombrero with his outfit. Jamie and this new friend in the room found that they enjoyed dancing together. Though they did not share the same language, they even managed to communicate their shared appreciation of jalapenos. The result was that the spirits of everyone in the room were elevated by the exchange.

Another time, Jamie entered the room of a family from the Middle East. No one in the family spoke English, so Jamie started to sing a song and dance to lift the spirit of the patient. Suddenly the whole family rose to their feet and everyone in the room danced to the music of the song. No one needed to speak to share the joy of the moment.

Jamie has developed some relationships with patients that have gone on for years. His exchanges with them are personal and familiar. For instance, with one boy who has a fascination with dinosaurs, Jamie always talks about archeological digs, paleontology and recent discoveries. Jamie gets as excited about dinosaurs as the patient.

Another teenage patient who often seemed to carry a chip on his shoulder about having to deal with his chronic disease also became a friend. When I was getting to know him, he did not have much use for me. Then one day when I went to see him, I let Jamie take my place at his bedside. Lo and behold, the patient's face brightened. Suddenly he was a playful child. That day sealed a relationship. One time when the patient had his cellphone with him, he even videotaped Jamie and told him he was going to make him famous by putting him on his Facebook page.

Then there was the girl who was refusing to take her medicine one day. Her nurse thought I might coax her into swallowing her pills. I tried. I must have stayed with her for an hour that day without succeeding. But the failure was not without positive result for the time spent that day established a relationship that continued for several years. When she met Jamie, she was delighted to discover that he loves to sing and dance. From then on they danced together any time she came to the hospital.

I discovered through these long-term relationships with patients that Jamie is a friend for all ages. He can capture the hearts of young and old, toddlers, school age children, teens and adults. Because of his attitude of sociability and inclusivity, he is a versatile partner to have at my side.

When Jamie enters the exchange, I slip into the background. He takes up the whole space between the patient and me and fills it in ways I cannot. He is masterful at eliciting everyone's response and building a sense of the little community in the room. He is uninhibited in his faith in imagined possibility. More often than not I am awed by what Jamie can accomplish to create relationship, enliven the sense of community, to brighten the experience of a patient's day, and to transform anxious anticipation and fear into gladness. Despite the mischievous edge he presents, Jamie's mission, as the song says, is to give his love away.

Chapter Six

Rupert: May Good Fortune Bless the Road You Wander

"Aiy, the work of transformin' in hospital takes many arts and many hands." So asserts Rupert, who has his hands and art in on that process of transformation, as we shall see. For the next patient we are about to visit had an uncomplicated appendectomy yesterday. She will be attended by Rupert.

Not long after I began at the hospital, I dreamed up many characters for my repertoire. Not all of them seemed to serve to the benefit of patients, but one that did was Rupert. Rupert is an Irish chimney sweep who sweeps patients clear of pain and toxins much as he once cleared chimneys of soot and tar. He first addressed abdominal pain in a patient and ever after he has continued to see patients who have appendicitis, have had an appendectomy, or are being evaluated for abdominal pain, though over the years he has broadened his practice to the treatment of other ailments, as well. Dr. Merryandrew calls him into service when he deems Rupert can best treat a patient.

In discussing the Shield of Light, I acknowledged the tensile space around the body of a patient and between the patient and me. One of the ways, we feel and talk about that space around the body is to identify it as an energy field. I know there are those who claim to see the energy around the bodies of others and there are some who practice the manipulation of energy around another's body as a healing modality. But other than knowing that such techniques do exist, I know nothing at all about the practices of energy manipulation. The origin of Rupert's practice has only the oblique connection to health care through the acknowledgement of energy around the body. His practice derives from a confluence of obscurities.

When I was teaching eleventh grade in high school, I taught Wolfram von Eschenbach's *Parzival,* which is a twelfth century version of one of the two great myths that originated after the Classical period in Western civilization, the other being *Faust.* On the surface, *Parzival* is a great romance of knighthood and courtship in the Middle Ages. As a myth combining Arthurian legend and the Grail legend, it is a narrative of soul transformation. Being a medieval narrative of soul transformation, it references the medieval art of alchemy, which attempted through dissolution and distillation to transform matter into spiritual substance and likewise, modeled transformation of the soul through dissolution and reconstitution. One day while browsing through a book of alchemical drawings in preparation for class, I came upon a drawing that seemed to give visual representation to many images in the narrative. On a ribbon-like banner that swept across the drawing was written an aphorism that seemed to encapsulate the trajectories of the journeys of the two knights, Parzival and Gawain, whose stories dominate the book. It read: "The fixed has been rendered volatile, the volatile has been rendered fixed." In regard to this medieval myth of soul development, the saying suggests that what is needed to restore balance in the psyche when there is imbalance. It is a formula for working toward balance when there is imbalance either in an area in which there is excessive volatility, frequent disruption or emotional turmoil or in an area in which there is frozen rigidity, hardened inflexibility or stubborn resistance to change.

By associative processes of the mind this obscure reference entered into the development of Rupert's practice. It is a common question when someone is hurting to ask, "Where is it hurting." As the question rightly implies, pain creates a physical fixation point. What Rupert intuited is that if he could move the pain from the point of fixation and sweep it along a route leading out of the body, the pain would be relieved. As the alchemical saying goes "the fixed has been rendered volatile," which is a good thing.

Yet as obvious as it may seem that a chimney sweep in a hospital might be engaged in some kind of sweeping, the practice of sweeping pain and toxins from patients might never have come to consideration or realization had a high school student of mine not given me the present of a special glue brush he found on a trip to the Netherlands. A glue brush is a bookbinder's tool. To receive a special glue brush as a gift from a student was not really as bizarre as it may sound. For at the school along with the regular semester classes for English, I taught intensive two or three week seminars on some of the classic books of the Western tradition, such as *The Odyssey*, Ovid's *Metamorphosis, Parzival, The Divine Comedy*, and Goethe's *Faust.* In each of the three or four seminar classes I taught for each grade level, I guided students to design beautiful handmade books into which to record their assignments for the seminar. So my students all had years of experience gluing beautiful cover paper to cardboard to create the hard cover of a handmade book. I never used the special glue brush I was given for the purpose for which it was designed. Instead it rested for several years in an honored place on the shelf of an antique bookcase in my study, until the day Rupert was looking for a symbol of his trade to bring with him to the hospital and fixed his eye upon the brush. It looks like a long-handled shaving brush for a giant, is well balanced and has a good heft to it. It pleased Rupert and he thought he could certainly incorporate it into his work in the hospital, so it went along with me.

With that little bit of indirect explanation, we can enter Brittany's room with Rupert.

Dr. Merryandrew: Good morning, Brittany. Are you feeling better than yesterday?
Brittany: I'm feeling better, but I'm sore. I have pain where the doctor took out my appendix.
Dr. Merryandrew: Well, I think I could take away some of your pain. Would you like that?
Brittany: How?
Dr. Merryandrew: Actually I don't do it myself. I have an assistant who takes pains away. I'll have him tell you how he can help you. His name is Rupert. He'll

be right here. (Dr. Merryandrew squats, opens his case, takes off his pork pie hat, and replaces it with an Irish wool cap. Rupert stands up with a brush in his hand and introduces himself with an Irish lilt in his speech.)

Rupert: Aiy, so Brittany you got a problem, have ya? Well, if you've got a problem, I've got a solution. But I have to tell ya, I ain't a doctor. You know what I am?

Brittany: A leprechaun?

Rupert: A leprechaun you think? No, I'm not a leprechaun. There's no pot of gold at the end of my rainbow… I tell you what I am. I'm a chimney sweep. You know what a chimney sweep is?

Brittany: A person who sweeps chimneys.

Rupert: Right you are. A genius are ya?… Well, I'll tell you about myself. How old are you?

Brittany: I'm twelve.

Rupert: Ah, I was your age… I was twelve years old when I started working as a chimney sweep in my old country. In my old country we cooked on our fires in our fireplaces. As smoke would go up the chimneys, it would leave soot and tar in the chimneys. If you leave it there, you know what can happen? It can catch fire, burn the whole house down. You can't have that, can you? So folks had to hire a little fella' like me — I was a little runt of a fella.' Folks had to hire a little fella' like me to go up on the tops of the houses and go down the chimney on a rope with a brush and a broom, scrubbing away, getting all the soot and tar out of the chimney. When I got down to the bottom, I'd sweep it out and throw it in the dust bin. Folks could start their fires again; do their cooking. I was a bit like Santa Claus, don't you know, going down the chimneys. I had a lot of work in those days because everybody cooked on their fires... Well, I tell you what happened. I was only working a year; thirteen years old I was when my brush wore out. I had to buy a new brush.

So I go down the alleyway in my town... to an old, old shop. I open the door. (Rupert mimes opening a door) Creeeeak! I go inside. I look around. First thing I find is this brush. (Rupert holds out the brush for inspection.) You ever seen a brush like that?... No, of course not, I'll tell you why, it's a magic brush. I didn't know it myself at the time. But there I am walking around the shop with the brush in my hand, you know, the way you do in a shop when you're seeing if there's anything else you'd like to buy. And folks in the shop start saying, "Wonderful." "That tickles." "I feel lovely." I start looking around. What's going on in this shop, I wonder, the Savior arrive or something? But it weren't that at all. It were me brush. A magic brush it is. I just wave it over folks and they start to feel better. It takes the pain and poison out of them... Well, I'll tell you what I did when I discovered it. I quit my job and went to work with the doctors in my old country, sweepin' the pains and the poisons outta' folks...

Then I crossed the pond. That's what they call the Atlantic Ocean in my old country. I came to America, to New York City, the city with the high buildings. I went to work with the doctors there, in some of the biggest hospitals in the world, New York Hospital, Bellevue, Sloan-Kettering, Mt. Sinai. Then I come down here to work with Dr. Merryandrew. And here I am at your bedside. And I'm going to work on you; take the pain and the poison out of you. Are you ready for that?... Good, we'll get started then.

I'll tell you how I do it. I just move my brush over you, sweeping as I go. You just lie there where you are. I do it same as I done with the chimneys, I start at the top and work on down sweeping the pain and the poison out of you. Here we go... Uh oh, you can't have anything crossed. You got to uncross your legs... That's better. No arms crossed, no fingers crossed. If you've got something crossed, I can't get through. Okay, here we go. I start over your head, just move slowly down over your body." (Rupert begins silently weaving the brush over the patient.)

In the silence, Rupert goes about his work with great concentrated intensity. The silence shifts the dynamic from the mode of storytelling to the act of treatment. Holding the silence is important to lend seriousness to the practice. When Rupert starts to speak again, he brings the patient into engagement with the treatment so that the patient feels she is participating in the process.

Rupert: I've got a special movement across your body as I move down. Do you see what kind of movement it is?
Brittany: A figure eight?
Rupert: Right. What's a figure eight lying on its side?
Brittany: Infinity?
Rupert: Right again, infinity…

Weaving in a motion approximating the sign of infinity over the body of the patient is a choice Rupert made simply to give the movement of the brush in the air above the patient a graceful solemnity. Calling it the sign of infinity endowed the magic brush with additional mystery and magic as if it gathered power from the infinite and eternity.

Rupert: Some folks say when the brush moves over them and they start to feel the pain and poison moving in the body, it hurts a bit, but it only hurts for a moment… I pay special attention over your belly where you had the operation. Make a few extra passes… There we go. Now we sweep it on down to your feet and out. Gather it up in a dust pan. And throw it in the dust bin. (Rupert goes over to the trash can, presses the pedal to open the lid and gestures as if to throw the contents of a dust pan into the trash. As he does this, he turns his back on the patient for a moment. Then he turns quickly, breaking the dynamic again out of the solemnity during the treatment. He crouches slightly near the trash can, as if to get some perspective at a slight distance to assess the effect of the treatment.)

There you are, you're all swept out… (Putting the brush back in the Magic Treasure Box, he approaches the bedside.) But we can't leave you like that. If we left you like that, you'd be an empty shell of a girl. (Turning to the parent in the chair beside the bed.) We can't leave her like that can we, Mom?

Mom: No. I wouldn't like that.

Rupert: We've got to get your fires burning again. I'll tell you what I'll do. I'll give you a little kindling of my own to start your fire. You ready? (Rupert makes a gesture with his two hands cupped together as if he is digging into his heart. Then he turns his cupped hands toward the patient as if he is offering what he is holding in his palms. He gently undulates his hands to simulate the beating of the heart.) Here you go. Take this and put it inside you. (He offers the contents of his cupped hands to the patient. The patient mimes taking something from him and thrusts her hands against her chest. Sometimes a patient thrusts her hand to her mouth as if to swallow what was given.) Good. Now I'll light it with a match, get your fire burning. (Rupert mimes striking a match and moves it toward the patient, then shakes it as if to put the match out.) I almost burned my finger on that match. (He moves toward the trash can, presses the pedal on the lid to open it and throws the match into the trash. Then he turns quickly and crouches more deeply this time.)

Look at you now. There's fire in your eyes. (Standing) Pretty soon that fire and warmth will go down to your fingers and down to your toes. You'll be glowing. There'll be a golden light around you. You'll look like a princess. Your friends will ask you, Brittany, when you went into the hospital you didn't look so good. Now look at you. You look like a princess. How did that happen? When they ask you, tell 'em it were me, Rupert, fixed you up. You remember that? Rupert, the chimney sweep… I'll tell you what I'll do for you. I'll give you a blessing from my old country, that's Ireland. It's got some secret words in it. Gaelic they are. I'll tell you what they mean Safe Journey. (Rupert begins to sing the blessing.)

Slan Abhaile Slan Abhaile
May your dreams come true
Slan Abhaile Slan Abhaile
I'll remember you

Now the party's coming to an end
It makes the heart grow fonder
May good fortune always be your friend
And bless the road you wander

Slan Abhaile Slan Abhaile
May your dreams come true
Slan Abhaile Slan Abhaile
I'll remember you[7]

There you go. You're gonna be fine, young lady. (Rupert squats down at the Magic Treasure Box and takes off his Irish cap. Dr. Merryandrew puts his pork pie hat back on his head. Squatting at the box, Dr. Merryandrew addresses Brittany.)

Dr. Merryandrew: Did Rupert fix you up, Brittany. Rupert's a fine therapist. (Standing) When he works on you, you start to feel better. He's worked on a lot of Dr. Saadya's patients and they all feel better quickly. You'll be fine. You look better already. (As Dr. Merryandrew is leaving, Dr. Saadya knocks and enters.)

Dr. Saadya: (Jokingly) Who is this nosy guy? Wherever I go, he is there. In my patients' rooms... in the ER. Next he'll show up in the OR... How are you, doctor? How's my patient?

Dr. Merryandrew: Brittany is doing wonderfully. I had my assistant, Rupert, treat her just now for her

post-operative pain. Thanks to your skill and Rupert's, we have a patient who is on the way to a swift recovery. Isn't that right, Brittany?
Dr. Saadya: How about this guy, Brittany? How are you doing?
Brittany: I'm feeling better. He's fun.

Though he does not give shots or prescribe tinctures or pilules to dissolve under the tongue, my assistant Rupert treats illness homeopathically. For Rupert's magic is based on what Sir James Frazer in his classic work of anthropology, entitled *The Golden Bough,* designated as the Law of Similarity, which he defines as a kind of metaphoric relation. According to Frazer's Law of Similarity "like produces like." Following the law of similarity, homeopathic magic assumes that an effect can be produced in one context through association with a similar effect produced in another context. For Rupert, the act of sweeping tar and soot out of a chimney can be compared with clearing pain and poison our of the body by sweeping. At the bedside of a patient, Rupert performs a ritual that includes the use of homeopathic magic. As he sweeps his magic brush slowly through lemniscates over the supine body of the patient from head to toe, a gesture that approximates the way he once swept chimneys clear of soot and tar, he works with concentrated attention to sweep pain and poison from the body to give the patient some relief. He commits himself seriously to the task and is sincere in his efforts on behalf of the patient. Of course, Rupert wears a red nose as he performs this magic ritual of healing. So I would not presume, as he does, that the magic he employs works upon the patient's physical being. But in many instances, I can affirm that Rupert's magic affects an attitudinal change in patients. Something seems to happen in the psyche of the patients to whom Rupert attends; a magical effect is wrought on the level of the soul.

And since there is some magical effect of Rupert's service, it would be presumptuous of me to argue against his curative claim. It may be that the attitudinal change to which I can attest does, in fact, indirectly influence the physical body of the patient. After all, body and soul are not so distinctly separate as portrayed in our mental constructs of them. We generally assume that what happens in the body affects the psyche. If we are ill, our mood is often also afflicted. So why could it not be the other way round? Yet as I raise the question, I have to disqualify myself from making any assertions regarding its answer. I do not have the medical background or experience for that though I know others much more qualified than me have had things to say in this regard.

Before I started in the hospital, I read Norman Cousins inspiring account in *Anatomy of an Illness as Perceived by the Patient: Reflections on Healing and Regeneration* of curing himself with a combination of self-confidence, emotional strength and humor. I also read his later account in *The Healing Heart: Antidotes to Panic and Helplessness* of refusing surgery and again adjusting his behavior to cure himself after congestive heart failure. And I looked into the research he did after he left his post as editor of *The Saturday Review* and spent ten years at the UCLA medical school researching the relationship between the mind and medicine in healing. Before coming to the hospital I also read Dr. Rachel Naomi Remen's beautifully told stories in *Kitchen Table Wisdom: Stories that Heal* and *My Grandfather's Blessings: Stories of Strength, Refuge and Belonging*, which demonstrate how the influences of positive emotional engagement and hope are not without physical effects. Her work with Commonweal impressed upon me just how much healing remains a mystery and part of the mystery is how much body and spirit are intertwined.

Not too long after I started in the hospital, my sister also introduced me to Dr. Lewis Mehl-Madrona's book, *Coyote Medicine: Lessons from Native American Healing.* Intrigued with how he integrates Western medicine with Native American storytelling and ritual practices, I continued to follow his work in *Narrative Medicine: The Use of History and Story in the Healing Process* and *Healing the Mind through the Power of Story: The Promise of Narrative Psychiatry.* He himself reports that there are those who consider him a shaman healer because he is so effective in the use of story and ritual with patients.

I mention these few from whom I have taken inspiration here. In their different ways they suggest to me that body and soul are more integrally aligned than we allow ourselves to assume. But I am sure there are others with whom I am not familiar who have entered into considerations of this kind in thought and practice, as well. So if I am not equipped to make a wise assessment, yet it is the sincere hope of a fool that such a little ritual of healing as Rupert performs might indeed serve in some measurable way in the process of healing.

But with as serious an attitude and with as true sincerity as Rupert maintains when he sees a patient, I would hope that the intercessory imagination of a fool might serve in its own right. It is with that belief that I return to the hospital each day. For I can positively affirm that imagination bestows flexibility and freedom of thought and feeling upon those it visits. It brings levity where there is heaviness of spirit. It breathes light into the darkness of uncertainty and fear. It stirs the will to leap in moments of despondency. It spurs the heart with hope in moments of despair.

Chapter Seven

The Grey Wolf's Wife

To reiterate what I have said earlier, story has a special province in the realm of imagination. For story is how we make meaning of life. As I said, we join the episodes of our lives as story into a vision of direction and destiny. Like the fragmented images of dreams, the events of our lives take order and significance when we weave them together in narration. We need stories to situate us in time and space, to awaken us to the wonders all around us, to plunge us into the flow of life and hold us in life's arrested moments, to enchant our daily reality and dazzle us with possibility, to enthrall us with the mystery of being. We tell stories for inspiration, guidance and solace, to define our identities as individuals and connect us as individuals in community with others. When we hear or tell a story and we are caught in the spell of narration, we know, as the old masters of story knew, that life is full of magic and miracle.

One day, I was thinking about how I needed a story to tell girls in the hospital who would not identify with the hunter in the tale of "The Golden Feather." It was a period in my time in the hospital when I was seeing a lot of girls ages nine and older. They were at a good age to attend to a long story. And as I visited with them, they seemed to move easily into the realm of imagination. I browsed through my volumes of Andrew Lang's nineteenth century anthology of folk and fairy tales. I was not quite sure what I was looking for in a story, but as I browsed I started to formulate criteria for what I wanted in a tale. First of all, I wanted the story to have a heroine. I did not want her to be passive. I wanted her to be a character who took initiative, who was bold and courageous, as well as caring and compassionate. I imagined her integrated with the cosmos and impassioned about the natural world. And as I read through old tales, I started to think that I would like to tell a story that would have both the mystique of the old fairy tales and an accessibility that would seem contemporary. That put me on the spot. I realized if I were going to try to meet my criteria, I would have to write a story of my own. "The Grey Wolf's Wife" is the result of those deliberations. When I started to write I did not worry about meeting all my criteria. Curiously, the story seemed to write itself in two quick spurts and I felt like I was recording what was dictated to me.

I remember the first patient to whom I told this story. She had been in the hospital for several days with pancreatitis. She was a quiet, thoughtful girl who always seemed to appreciate it when I walked into her room to break up the medical routines of the day. As I began to narrate, she grew quiet and still and listened intensely. I had to pause for one interruption, but she wanted to get right back to the story. Near the end, her nurse came into the room to get her out of bed for a walk down the hall. I finished the telling, she got out of bed, and I joined them as they began their walk. I heard the nurse ask her, What was that story about? She responded, it was complicated, and left it at that. Yet in the reflective way she said, it was complicated, I got the sense that she was integrating it into her being and I was reassured. I have told "The Grey Wolf's Wife" a number of times since then.

Today, Natalie is a patient whom I believe would enjoy this story. She is ten years old. She has been here for several days while the team of doctors and residents have tried to figure out her diagnosis. For all that, she has a very positive attitude. She seems to have a patient thoughtful perspective on her predicament. Some children whine and start to complain after several days of diagnostic tests. But Natalie takes it all in stride. She always seems to welcome what I come up with for her.

Dr. Merryandrew: Good morning, Natalie. How are you today?... Yesterday, you told me you like stories, so I'm going to tell you a story today. Is this a good day to hear a story?... Good, OK. But I have to tell you before I get started…all my stories are old stories whether they are about things that happened long ago or things that happened yesterday. They are old stories because I learned from the old masters. The old masters knew that life was full of magic and miracle. They knew that animals could turn into people and people could turn into animals; that any path goes down before it goes up and it goes through darkness before it comes to light. They knew we meet many guides and helpers in our lives. Some of these are guides we seek. Some are helpers who show up when we think we are lost, stuck and alone. Sometimes they help us by doing what we ask. Sometimes they guide us by asking us to do something for them. Maybe if we listen to the old stories, we will know what the old masters knew. Maybe if more people hear the old stories, there will be more people around who know that life is full of magic and miracle.

Not long ago, but not so recently either, there was a girl, not too old, but not too young either. She lived with her mother and father on a farm. In the afternoon when her chores were finished, she would go out into the field to feed the birds. She was grateful to the little songbirds whose songs accompanied her in the morning when she went early to her chores. She loved the swallows and the robins and the sparrows. She would sing to them as she fed them in the afternoon. Her father called her Sparrow because she sang so sweetly as she fed the birds.

But when the black crows came to the field in the afternoon to be fed with the other birds, Sparrow shooed them away. "None for you," she shouted at them.

One day when Sparrow went to the field in the afternoon, a man dressed in the clothes of the forest people came walking out of the woods beside their farm. He was cradling a small animal in his arms.

"Sparrow," the man addressed her.

"How did you know to call me that?" she asked. He did not answer her.

Here in the story, a character does not answer a question asked. Although this is the only instance where a question arising in the story is explicitly left unanswered, there are other places in the story where questions arise and go unanswered. Quite deliberately the narrative does not explain moments that seem inexplicable. As unanswered questions accumulate in the story, I hope listeners start to sense that the narrative is playing at the border of mystery. Mystery yields no answers. It commands our reverence and awe.

"Sparrow, will you raise this wolf cub? He has lost his mother and will die if he is not taken in."

Sparrow thought the grey wolf cub looked like a puppy and she loved him right off. So she said she would. The man gave her the cub and without another word turned and went back into the forest.

Sparrow raised the cub and because she was a gentle and caring girl, he was gentle too. Every day they ran together through the field beside the forest. Now and then, the wolf would stop where the man had brought him out of the woods and stare into the trees as if he heard someone calling. But Sparrow would always put her hand on him and coax him back to the fields and farm.

As wolves grow quickly, soon he was full grown and ran silently like the wind. At a short distance, he could sprint faster than a horse and he liked to run. At night when the distant forest was alive with the howling of wild wolves, her wolf would wake in her room where he slept, go to the open window and look out at the distance across the field. But he was always settled beside her when she woke in the morning to do her early chores. They would go out together and listen to the chorus of the songbirds each morning.

Sparrow loved the companionship of the grey wolf. He had become her partner and friend in everything. He did not avert his eyes like wild animals do even when they have been raised in domestic circumstances. He held her gaze when she looked at him and she often found him watching her like a protector when they were doing something in the field or the forest. Once he pulled her away from a copperhead snake when Sparrow was bringing wood in from the woodpile. Another time on a mountain, he caught her when she slipped on a rock ledge and would have fallen hundreds of feet into a chasm. There was something in her grey wolf's eyes when he looked at her that seemed almost human.

Then one day in the fall of the year when Sparrow and her wolf were running through the fields, the grey wolf stopped at the old spot by the woods and listened again. As she kept running, Sparrow called him to come, but he didn't seem to hear her. She turned around. He was looking directly at her. Later she could not remember whether he looked like he was saying goodbye or like he was calling her to follow him. The next instant, he turned and darted into the woods at the place where the man had brought him out of the woods.

Sparrow ran after him. She ran and ran but he was faster and could more easily run through the brush and trees of the forest. Soon it grew dark in the forest and Sparrow could not see where her wolf went. She realized she had followed him deep into the forest and would have to wait where she was over night or she would lose her way wandering in the dark.

In the morning when she woke in the woods, Sparrow did not recognize where she was. But as the sun rose, she walked deeper into the forest in the direction away from the rising sun. She knew the farm was the other way, so her wolf must have been going away from the farm. About noon, when the sun was high overhead, she came to a small hut in the woods. She approached it to see if there was anyone to speak to in the hut. When she rapped at the door, the door swung open and Sparrow went inside. Inside an old woman, wrapped in a shawl, sat in a rocking chair by the hearth.

"I am looking for my grey wolf, mother. Have you seen my grey wolf?" Sparrow asked.

"Come closer, dear. I am Mother Wind. I have been out in the forest all through the night, but I have not seen your grey wolf. But if you will do me a service, I will send you to someone who may know where your grey wolf is. Could you bring me the first leaf that fell in the Fall. I want it for my leaf collection. Find that leaf and I will help you on your way."

Sparrow went out of the hut. Many leaves were drifting from the branches of the forest to the ground and many more were already spread over the ground. How would she ever find the one that had fallen first, she thought. She sat down on the edge of the well in Mother Wind's yard and started to cry.

"Why are you crying, child?" asked a very old turtle at her feet.

"What? Oh, it is you who asked." Sparrow looked down at Old Turtle. "I am looking for my grey wolf. Mother Wind said she will help me find him if I find the first leaf that fell in the Fall. But I don't know how I will ever do that. There are so many leaves down already. How could I know the first?"

"I think I can help you if you will pick me up so I can sit beside you," said Old Turtle. "That's better; now I don't have to scream. Well, I saw the first leaf fall in the well when Mother Wind was blowing through the forest last week. Lower me into the well and I will bring it up for you."

Sparrow lowered Old Turtle into the well and brought him up again. When he came up, he was holding a brown leaf that looked like any water-logged leaf you might find under water. Sparrow took it from him. When she held it in her hand in the sun, it suddenly turned red, then gold, then all colors of the rainbow.

"Oh, Old Turtle, look at the leaf. How wonderful it is," Sparrow said. "How can I thank you?"

"Never mind that," said Old Turtle. "Just put me back down on the ground and I will be on my way."

After she said goodbye to Old Turtle, Sparrow ran inside with the leaf for Mother Wind.

"You have done well, dear. Now I will tell you who may know where your grey wolf is. Follow the path that leads behind my cottage until you come to the meadow beside the stream from where you can see the mountains rising in the distance. There is a giant pine tree there. Climb to the top of the pine and call to Sister Cloud from there. If she is not in a dark mood, she will come down to speak with you and she may be able to tell you where your grey wolf is.

"Now here, dear, take this whistle with you as a gift from me. I am sure the path ahead for you will be difficult and dangerous, but you are a brave girl and can master by yourself most of the challenges you will face. But if there ever comes a time when all seems lost, your life is threatened, and you can imagine no escape, blow this whistle. I will hear it wherever you are and I will send one of my offspring to help you."

The giant pine was just where Mother Wind said it would be. The branches started low to the ground and Sparrow climbed easily to the top as if she were climbing a ladder. At the top, she called to Sister Cloud.

"Sister Cloud, have you seen my grey wolf?" she called to the sky.

"Grey, indeed. These are indeed grey dark days for I have lost my most beautiful jewels. And what have you lost, dear, that you come bothering me when I have lost something most precious to me?" said Sister Cloud.

"I have lost my dear grey wolf. I raised him from when he was a cub and he has been my companion and friend. Then suddenly he ran off into the forest and I cannot find him," said Sparrow.

"Did you do something to drive him off?" asked Sister Cloud.

"No, I swear I did not," said Sparrow.

"Well, I don't know. Maybe if you help me find the precious jewel necklace I have lost, I can help you," said Sister Cloud. "The last time I remember that I had my necklace, I was in the mountains."

Out of the tree, Sparrow looked up at the peak and started to climb the mountain. There was no trail and the way was hard. She saw nothing that looked like jewels or a necklace. When she grew tired from the climb, she rested. But she had not rested long when jays on the branches beside her in the mountain forest cried out, "Higher."

When she got to a knoll at the edge of the tree line, Sparrow rested again. This time a red-tailed hawk high overhead called to her, "Higher." She climbed until she *reached the rocky summit. Still no necklace of jewels. She sat down on a rock too tired to cry. As she sat, she watched a spider go in and out of a crevice in the rock. As she watched him go in and out over and over, she began to think he was doing his little dance for her. Maybe he wanted her to look where he disappeared into the rock each time. When she tried to look for him, she saw what looked like a little patch of snow. She thought the snow must not have melted in the sun because it was hidden under the cover of the rocks. But as she looked more closely, she saw that what she thought was a shining patch of snow was really a chain of white gold in which were set amethysts, sapphires and topaz. This, she thought, must be Sister Cloud's jewel necklace.*

"Sister Cloud, Sister Cloud, I have found it," she screamed to the sky.

Still dark with gloom, Sister Cloud came hurtling toward her from a ways away, descended like a mist over the mountain peak, gathered up her necklace and then lifted, opened and brightened into a smile. "And what did you say I can do for you?" asked Sister Cloud.

"I have lost my grey wolf. Can you help me find my grey wolf?" answered Sparrow.

"Oh, I see," said Sister Cloud. "No, I am sorry I cannot help you. I have not seen your grey wolf. You must really go ask Sister Moon. She sees more than me. If you go down to the shallow ford in the stream that

runs through the valley, you will find the path of light that leads to Sister Moon. Follow the path through the ford and beyond and it will lead you to Sister Moon. Be brave and prosper. And thank you for finding my necklace. I will remember that."

That night Sparrow crossed the ford on the path of moonlight and kept following it on the other side of the stream. As she walked in the light, she felt the land to the right and left of her drop away. She sensed she was suspended high in the air on a ridge of light, bordered on either side by chasms of darkness. Cold air from either side brushed her skin. Behind her there was a buzzing and whirring as if an army of wasps or stinging demons were swarming after her. She started to run, keeping her feet on the light so she did not slip into the abyss that opened on either side. Then suddenly she stopped. There in front of her, blocking her progress, stood a darkly robed giant with the hood on his robe pulled up so it hid his face... if he had a face. In his hands there was a club that looked as thick as an uprooted tree trunk with a boulder lodged in its roots. He heaved the club up over his head, preparing to strike.

Sparrow turned back toward the swarming mass of stinging demons. As she turned, on the back of her neck she felt the giant's hot breath. She smelled its sour odor. Sparrow was alone, stuck, and terrified. Then she remembered the whistle that Mother Wind had given her. She reached in her cloak, found the whistle and blew a long loud blast above the noise of the buzzing swarm behind her. The whistle blast sounded shrill. Then as it drifted into the dark, Sparrow was lifted gently on an up-draft of wind. She sailed over the hooded menace and was set down again further along on the path of light. Fearing for her life, she ran until she nearly crashed into the shining gates of the palace of the moon. They opened for her and then closed again as soon as she passed over the threshold. In a room that smelled like a Spring river flooded with melted snow and ice, Sister Moon sat on her shining silver throne.

Sparrow knelt down the way she thought you are supposed to do when you come before royalty and said, "Sister Moon, I am looking for my grey wolf. Have you seen my grey wolf?"

"Stand up please. No need to kneel in my presence. I have been watching you on your journey, Sparrow. You are a brave girl to come through the perils of the path of my light. I think you will find your grey wolf. But I have not seen him yet in the course of my monthly journey. I am sorry, Sparrow. You must journey beyond me to Father Sun. Only he can tell you where your wolf may be. It is a difficult path to Father Sun. Stay alert. If you fail to concentrate for an instant along the way you will be in grave danger.

"Here, take this dark mirror. Only with a dark reflecting glass can you find the path to the Sun from here. When you step outside my palace through the gates by which you entered, turn around immediately or you will be blinded. Face the gate again. Then hold up the looking glass until you can see a golden light shining in the center. Walk backward holding the glass and keep the golden light in the center. The glass will be your compass guide. So long as you keep the golden light in the center, nothing will happen to you. But if your mind drifts and you let the light slide away from the center, there will be danger for you. Go directly and safe journey, Sparrow."

Sparrow did as she was instructed by Sister Moon and kept the golden light in the center of the glass as she went. Several times, she caught herself when her mind started to drift. But then somewhere along the way as she walked backward while staring at the reflection in the glass, her foot hit a snag. She tottered and almost fell. The glass slipped from her hand and started to fall away from her as if it were flying weightlessly into space. She leapt to retrieve it and she too began to float weightless in space. She caught the handle of the mirror just before she started spinning and spinning head-over-heels through what seemed like endless darkness. She clutched the glass, but it was no use trying to look for the golden light in it. Had she remembered it, she could not have reached for her whistle as she was spinning. Nor could she have caught her breath to blow a blast on it. She was hurtling uncontrollably through darkness.

But as she spun uncontrollably, Sparrow found a quiet harmony in the spinning. It was as if she were in the center of a protective cloud where she felt no difference between inside and outside herself. Even though she was spinning it seemed to her that she was absolutely still. And then for no reason of her own, she said to herself, "Sparrow is flying to her nest in a storm."

As soon as she said that, she stopped spinning, and landed on her feet in a dazzlingly bright garden ringed all round with sunflowers. The gardener came toward her with a spade in his hand and said in a gentle tone, "Don't step on the cabbages, child."

"Father Sun?" asked Sparrow.

"Yes, Sparrow, how can I help you?" Father Sun asked.

"Oh, Father Sun, I have lost my grey wolf. He ran away and I want to beg him to come back to me. I went to Mother Wind, Sister Cloud and Sister Moon to ask if they had seen where he went, but they had not. Father Sun, can you help me find my grey wolf?"

"You have shown courage, little Sparrow, to have flown so far in pursuit of your grey wolf. Now you must go home and wait. Wait for him to return. Go

home and feed the birds again, little Sparrow. And do not shoo the crows away. The crows are my messengers. Be generous with them and they will tell you when your grey wolf is coming.

"Here, I will give you some seeds from my garden to grow a garden for yourself so you will always have sunlight in your garden."

Father Sun gave Sparrow a little pouch in which he poured sunflower seeds from his garden. He hung the pouch on a silk ribbon and tied the ribbon around Sparrows neck so that she would not lose it on her journey home. When it was tied around her neck, Sparrow seemed aglow with sunlight. Then Father Sun twirled her around and sent her down to earth on a sunbeam where she landed an instant after she left his garden. She was home.

Sparrow returned to feeding the songbirds in the afternoon. But as Father Sun suggested, she also fed the crows. A year and a day from the time her grey wolf ran away, crows in a great cluster made a tremendous commotion in the oak branches where the grey wolf had entered the woods and the man had brought Sparrow the wolf cub before that. Sparrow looked up to see if the crows were yammering about a hawk in the forest. But they were not circling anything in the trees. Then what was all the commotion about? Sparrow ran to see.

Out of the woods came a man dressed in the clothes of the forest people. He was a ruggedly handsome man. He walked with a remarkable grace as if he were gliding soundlessly over the ground the way a wolf moves. As he came toward her, Sparrow immediately recognized something familiar in his eyes.

"Sparrow," he said, "are you ready to come with me?"

"Yes," she said, "Yes, I am ready, my Grey Wolf."

I have heard some people say when Sparrow said yes, they both turned into wolves and disappeared into the forest. Others have said they lived as human beings in a simple cottage in the forest where all the animals and birds served them and they never lacked for anything. Outside their cottage was a luxurious garden ringed by sunflowers that bloomed all year round. If Sparrow gave you seeds from her sunflowers to eat, you were assured of good fortune for a year and a day. The story of their lives together, however, will have to be told in another tale for another day's telling.

All I can say now is that Sparrow's mother and father told me she visited them regularly. And when she came, she and her children carried themselves with the grace of Nature and always spoke to them of wondrous things.

That's my story for you today, Natalie. Did you like it?... You know each time you hear one of the old

stories, you can put yourself into it in a different place in the story. One time you may feel it would be thrilling to have the companionship of a wild animal like a wolf. Another time you may feel as if a dear friend has disappeared and you want to go searching for her. Sometimes you may feel you are given an impossible task to complete. Then there are the times in your life that it seems magical agents show up to help you. Every time you hear the story, it becomes new.
Natalie: That was a good story. I liked it.

I had the good fortune to know and learn from Thomas Berry during the last years of his life. Thomas was a Passionist priest, a world renown eco-theologian, and a prophet of what he called the coming "Ecozoic Age," when human beings will live in mutually enhancing relationship with all other beings in the Earth community, with the flowers and the trees and the grasses, the insects, the bees and the butterflies, the squirrels and the rabbits, the chipmunks, the bear and the deer, the lions and the leopards and the antelopes, the fish and the birds. Thomas wrote in his seminal book, *The Dream of the Earth,* "Children need a story that will bring personal meaning together with the grandeur and meaning of the universe..."[8] When I wrote the story of "The Grey Wolf's

Wife," I had those words of Thomas as a beacon of guidance. When he wrote *The Dream of the Earth*, however, Thomas had in mind that children need to hear the scientific story of the evolving of the universe, which he felt is the new myth of creation for our current period of history. I had no intention to tell the story of the evolving universe to a patient in the hospital. But I did want to create some sense of intimacy with the vastness of the universe in the story.

There is an apocryphal story told of Albert Einstein in which the great scientist of the 20th century recommends fairy tales to a woman who inquires of him how to educate her son. According to several different investigators, the original account of this story, which could never be verified, first appeared in a publication of the Montana State Library in 1958. Here is the original mention as cited by Maria Popova in her blog entitled, *The Marginalian.*

> In the current *New Mexico Library Bulletin*, Elizabeth Margulis tells a story of a woman who was a personal friend of the late dean of scientists, Dr. Albert Einstein. Motivated partly by her admiration for him, she held hopes that

her son might become a scientist. One day she asked Dr. Einstein's advice about the kind of reading that would best prepare the child for this career. To her surprise, the scientist recommended 'Fairy tales and more fairy tales.' The mother protested that she was really serious about this and she wanted a serious answer; but Dr. Einstein persisted, adding that creative imagination is the essential element in the intellectual equipment of the true scientist, and that fairy tales are the childhood stimulus to this quality.[9]

I cannot say that I was specifically thinking about the advice to a mother attributed to Einstein when I was writing my own story, but recognition of the importance of creative imagination pervades everything I do. The wisdom encapsulated in the advice motivates me to tell fairy tales in the hospital. So Einstein's words were certainly in the back of my mind as I wrote "The Grey Wolf's Wife."

On the combined advice of two luminaries of the 20th century, I began to write my modest tale. As you can see, it became a fairytale about a human and her mutually-enhancing relationships in community with beings of the more than human world.

Much of what I do in the hospital is improvisational and interactive. As I have mentioned in relation to the Shield of Light, often in lieu of verbal exchange, interaction takes place as reverberation in the tension of the space between the patient and me and is a visceral experience. This is the nature of the interaction as Rupert sweeps his brush over a patient's body. Telling a story, however, is not interactive. That does not mean that telling a story is not relational. As I have said earlier, much like telling a bedtime story to a child, it is my experience that the one-to-one connection engaged while telling a story to one patient in a hospital room is intensely relational. Telling a story is a significantly different sharing than reading a story to a child. Moment by moment I assess the patients response. I adjust my pace to the indications of attentiveness in the patient's eyes. I make more subtle adjustments as I sense where the patient is internally moved. I will then fill the words with more feeling and intensity. These are adjustments human beings make with each other when we meet face-to-face though we would be hard pressed to identify how that inner harmonizing takes place as we relate. Yet we sense the tone and rhythm of the inner music of another and the tone and rhythm of our own inner music shifts.

In truth, if I do not feel the potential for that inner synchronization with a patient, I will usually choose not to tell a long story. When I try to override that inclination, I usually find the telling labored. But when the potential is there to offer a story, I think of the telling of a story as an intravenous infusion from Dr. Merryandrew's pharmacopeia. I attribute to the patient the experience I have in hearing a good story. For a good story goes right to the heart of my being where meaning and identity reside, where I feel centered and at peace, the place where I feel connected with the source of life and inspiration, the place, too, from which my sense of well-being radiates. Every good story stirs me to reflect on motivation and character, values and relations in my own life. As I say to patients, these old stories, full of twists and turns and transformations, cause me to consider how I respond to where I am with myself in any moment of my life. They are powerful medicine for the soul. The time has to be right for the patient in order for me to tell a long story like "The Grey Wolf's Wife." When the time is right, telling a story creates a powerful relation.

Chapter Eight

Jamie II: It Wouldn't Be Make-believe If You Believed

If storytelling holds verbal interaction to a minimum, by contrast, Jamie is always an engaging interlocutor. He thrives on dialogue. Even with the most taciturn he likes to get a conversation going. Over time he has developed his own repertoire to draw patients into verbal interaction.

We just watched a patient named Jordan, age seven years, be shown into an emergency room. He was quiet and seemed shy. Jamie may have to draw him out.

Jamie: Hi, Jordan. I'm Jamie. This is my dad, Dr. Merryandrew.
Jordan: Hi.
Jamie: Can I sing you a song? I'll sing you my theme song.

It's only a paper moon
sailing over a cardboard sea,
but it wouldn't be make-believe
if you believed in me.

It's only a canvas sky
hanging over a muslin tree,
but it wouldn't be make-believe
if you believed in me.

Without your love
it's a honky-tonk parade.
Without your love
it's a melody played in a penny arcade.

It's a Barnum and Bailey world
just as phony as it can be.
But it wouldn't be make-believe
if you believed in me.[10]

Jamie searched around for a song of introduction and struck on "Paper Moon." Adults might think that it shows a certain self-consciousness that he chose "Paper Moon" as his theme song, but he does not sing it with any irony. Children never seem to snicker at what we adults might think has a touch of irony.

My sense is that children under nine years old do not pick up on the possible irony of Jamie singing "Paper Moon." One of the things I noticed during the four years of research I did for my dissertation on the storytelling of children ages eight to twelve was that until the age of nine the boundary between the world of imagination and what we adults call the world of reality is very porous. As we saw with Natasha earlier, a delightful example of the expression of the porous nature of the boundary between imagination and reality is how without being self-conscious at all, a child will argue with Jamie about whether or not he is real. During the years of my dissertation research, I found that children eight years old would freely launch into telling an elaborate imaginary tale without the slightest provocation and with the greatest alacrity. They made little distinction between a story told by a child about an event from yesterday with her peers and a fantasy about a cat that says "I don't know all the time." They may "know a hawk from a handsaw," as truth and falsehood were distinguished by Hamlet, but for young children before the age of nine it seems, a story is a story is a story.

And a song is a song is a song, and it is to be assessed as a melody that is or is not enjoyed.

Jamie sings "Paper Moon" as it was written and as it has been sung by such artists as Nat King Cole, as a serenade. With the purity of his intention, Jamie reveals that beneath his tough and sassy facade, he is really a sentimental romantic. He believes every patient he meets is beautiful and good and comes into the world with a special gift. It is the beauty of the music of the song to which the patients respond.

When he finishes singing, often the simple beauty of the tune evokes a compliment or an offer to sing a song in response. Sometimes when a child does not freely offer Jamie a song, to get interaction going, Jamie will make the request for one.

Jordan: That was a nice song.
Jamie: Thank you, Jordan. Now you sing me a song.
Jordan: I don't know… What are you wearing on your arm?
Jamie: It's my name bracelet. You have a bracelet with your name on it and so do I. My Dad has a badge with his picture and name on it. See?… Don't you want to sing me a song?

The Pediatric Unit is enlightened enough to have a playroom for patients. The recreational therapist is a talented young woman from whom I have learned a great deal. She keeps the playroom well stocked with arts and crafts supplies, as well as games and toys. She also gives patients as much guidance as they need in the use of the materials. She herself is accomplished in all the arts and crafts she supplies. One day in the playroom during bead crafting, a patient made Jamie a bead bracelet small enough for his arm out of elastic cord and alphabet beads. Jamie put it on his right wrist and has worn it ever since.

Jordan: Mom, what should I sing?
Mom: Why don't you sing a song from church.
Jordan: I think I'll sing "Twinkle Twinkle…"

Church songs and "Twinkle Twinkle Little Star" are popular with many young children. Sometimes, too, mother's will join in for a duet of a contemporary popular song from a Disney movie like "Lion King" or "Frozen."

Jamie: That was beautiful, Jordan. Do you want to sing me another song?… No… OK… Tell me, what do you like to do when you aren't here?
Jeanine: Well, I like to play hide 'n seek.
Jamie: OK, let's play hide 'n seek. Close your eyes and I'll hide… OK, you can open your eyes now. (Jamie

removes himself from view by dropping on the side of the bed below the height of the mattress. Of course, the strings that support him are still held in plain sight.)
Jordan: I found you.
Jamie: Now you hide. (Jordan pulls the covers over his head.)
Jamie: Where's Jordan? Is he under the bed?... No... Is he behind Mom's chair?... No... Wait. Did I see something move under the covers? (Jordan throws the covers off.)
Jordan: You found me.

This little game of Hide 'n Seek that Jamie plays to draw children out has reminded me of something too easily forgotten when we cross the moat from childhood to adulthood. Playing the game again, I have been reminded that the true pleasure of Hide 'n Seek comes at the moment of being found. A child who steals into a hiding place where he cannot be found can all too easily start to feel abandoned or lost, as if the game goes on without him and he has been passed over. Watching children in the neighborhood around my house play Hide 'n Seek recently has confirmed this observation. Sometimes a child gets a hiding place that is never searched by the one who is "It" though the child is in plain view to me sitting in my yard across the street. If the child is not found after a brief time, he will steal out to a more obvious hiding place to be assured of being found. The neighborhood children squeal with delight when they are found, as does the one who finds them. I mention this quality of Hide 'n Seek to affirm that when Jamie and a patient play Hide 'n Seek in a hospital room, the game still has legitimacy. But it is hard to sustain it for long. So Jamie has other means of drawing a child into interaction.

Jamie: Jordan, do you see that flower in my hat? Do you know what it is?
Jordan: A daffodil?

In North Carolina, the daffodils of spring are abundant. Since the flower in Jamie's hat is yellow, it is a good guess to identify it is as a daffodil.

Jamie: It's yellow like a daffodil, but it's not a daffodil. It's just a little flower that grows in the grass. Do you know a flower like that?
Jordan: Ummm… I don't know.
Jamie: It's a dandelion.

I always find it surprising that so few young children guess "dandelion" when Jamie gives them the clue that his yellow flower is little and grows in the grass. Dandelions were so very much a part of my childhood but do not seem to be for children today. What I have found in the hospital corroborates what others have discovered, as well. In fact, in 2007, "dandelion" was actually dropped from the new edition of the Oxford Junior Dictionary. It was among forty words having to do with the natural world that were removed from the dictionary because children no longer use them enough to claim a space there. Words common to users of the computer, such as attachment, blog, bullet point, and such replaced them. Robert Macfarlane, a contemporary naturalist writer in England, and Jackie Morris, an artist and illustrator of children's books, created a wonderful book of poetic spells and illustrations of the words removed from the dictionary, called *The Lost Words*. It was their book that brought this little known fact to my attention. As I mentioned at the beginning of this day just before entering the Pediatric unit, I spend a lot of time in the natural world and think of myself as an advocate of time in childhood spent in relationship with the natural world. So I am glad that Jamie is doing his part to preserve "dandelion" in the vocabulary of children he sees and in their consciousness of the natural world.

Jamie: Have you ever picked up one of those little puff balls growing in the grass and made a wish on it? Those puff balls are dandelion seeds.

Jordan: Oh yeah, I did that. It didn't happen though.

Jamie: Maybe you just haven't waited long enough for it to happen… I'm going to tell you a secret about the dandelions when they are little yellow flowers growing in the grass, like the one I have in my hat. At night, when your mom is sleeping, the dandelions wake up and turn into real lions. They go roar through the neighborhood. ROAR! But the secret is, they are friendly lions. That's why they are called, "DANDY-LIONS." If you wake up in the night when everyone in your house is sleeping and you go to the window, you can see the dandelions out there. If you call to them, one will come to your window. You can jump on his back and he will take you off to Wonderworld. In Wonderworld there are kings and queens, princes and princesses, and knights and unicorns and rainbows. And you can do anything you would like to do in Wonderworld. If you went to Wonderworld, what would you like to do?

Jordan: I'd like to visit with my grandma.

Jamie: Is your grandma your favorite person?

Jordan: Yes. But my grandma died.

Children sometimes speak so freely of intimate things. Often in conversation with

Jamie, a child will reveal something deeply felt. In mentioning his grandmother's death, Jordan does not so much express his sadness at his loss of his grandma, as he does the love and appreciation and attachment he still feels in relation to his grandma. In a way that adults cannot fully grasp, children very naturally and intuitively know that love does not end with loss. Love continues to connect Jordan with his grandma. Jordan's love for his grandma bridges the span between here and beyond.

Just as the boundary between true stories and fantasies is porous for young children, the boundary separating a child from a relative who has died can be freely crossed. These seem to be characteristics of the culture of childhood that define childhood as very different than adulthood. We forget, just as we forget in the game of Hide 'n Seek that the pleasure comes from being found, we forget how different it is to live in the culture of childhood, which we adults have left behind. But Jamie has not forgotten.

Jamie: I'm sorry, Jordan. Tell me about your grandma.
Jordan: Grandma used to take care of me when my momma had to go to work. She would take me to the park and push me on the swings. Then we'd go home

and she would let me help her in the kitchen. Grandma made the best mac and cheese and the best chocolate chip cookies and pudding. And sometimes in the afternoon, after lunch, I would sit on the couch with grandma and we would look at the comics in the newspaper. Grandma would read them to me and show me the words and that's how I learned to read.

Jamie: It sounds like your grandma was very special.

Jeanine: She was. You know what? When I went to school, I didn't have to have the teacher teach me reading because grandma taught me to read. And she taught me my numbers too.

Children move seamlessly from deep feeling back into full participation in the present moment. They pass back through the porous boundary between beyond and here. Jamie is alert to the shift.

Jamie: Do you know how to count?

Jordan: Of course.

Jamie: I can only count to four, that's all. One… (Jamie raises his right arm)… Two…(Jamie raises his right leg)… Three… (Jamie raises his left arm)… Four… (Jamie raises his left leg)… That's it. It's enough, don't you think? What do you need all those numbers for? What can you do with them?

Jordan: That's silly. You can do all kinds of things with numbers. You can count things. You can add. You can count how many cookies are left on the cookie plate.
Jamie: Oh, that sounds good. I like cookies.
Jordan: I'll teach you to count.
Jamie: I showed you I can only count to four. See… One (right arm)… Two (right leg)… Three (left arm)… Four (left leg)… That's it.
Jordan: You can count your head as five. And your hat as six. And your flower as seven. And your banana as eight. (Jamie has a banana shaped button sewn to the right side of his overalls) And your… What is that thing? (Jamie has a polka dotted cloth hanging from one pocket of his overalls.)
Jamie: It's my handkerchief.
Jordan: And your handkerchief as nine. And your whole self as ten. Yay! Now you can count to ten. After ten, it's easy.
Jamie: Let me try. One… Two… Three… Four… My head… Five… My hat… Six… My flower… Seven… My banana… Eight… My handkerchief… Nine… My whole self… Ten… Yay! I did it… Oh, who's that?... Oh, Hi, Dr. Jefferson. Guess what, Dr. Jefferson, Jordan taught me to count to ten. Isn't that great? He's a great teacher.
Dr. Jefferson: That's great, Jamie. But didn't you tell me you were twelve? Shouldn't Jordan have taught you to count to twelve?

Jamie: Uh oh, Jordan, what are we going to do?
Jordan: Your name bracelet can be eleven and your red nose can be twelve. There!
Jamie: Bracelet eleven, red nose twelve. There, Dr. Jefferson, I'm red nose. Ooops! I'm twelve. See, Jordan is a good teacher. Maybe we should keep him around so he can teach me other things.
Dr. Jefferson: I'm not sure Jordan's mom would like that, Jamie.
Mom: It would be fine with me if you just get him to feeling better. Anyway, he says he wants to be a doctor. Maybe you could show him what it's like.
Dr. Jefferson: Well, Jordan, let's see what's going on for you so we can get you on the way to becoming a doctor.
Jamie: Thanks, Jordan. I'll remember everything you taught me. My head – five, my hat – six, my flower – seven, my banana – eight, my handkerchief – nine, my whole self – ten, my bracelet – eleven, my red nose – twelve.

Boundaries in Jamie's world are as porous as they are in the world of children. He easily passes between reality and imagination and back without a pause. But unlike children, Jamie weaves between the worlds of children and adults, between patients and doctors and nurses and families as if there are no boundaries or different spheres of life. For Jamie we are all one unified community of equals. As he weaves between the families, patients, doctors, and nurses, with enthusiasm for the life of each patient, Jamie weaves between illness and health and restores patients like Jordan to a sense of well-being.

Chapter Nine

Harmonies of Healing

It is a wonderful feature of the Pediatric Emergency Department in our hospital that there are decorations around the department and that the decorations follow the theme of flight. There are biplane and helicopter lights over the desk at the nurses' station. A model of a small prop-plane is fixed on a wall near one entrance. Best of all, the one free wall in each patient room in the department is painted with a mural based around the theme of flight. There is a beach scene with kites flying. There are skies full of air balloons. There is one room where the mural depicts an astronaut out from a space module for a walk in space. And in this room we are about to enter, there are planets and stars and nebulae viewed from a spaceship that is suggested by a view of its control panel pictured in the far corner of the mural near the entrance door to the room. Each one of the murals inspires imagination to take flight.

This room we are about to enter has a special appeal for me because I love to look up at the stars and planets at night. I watch the passage of the seasons through the zodiac and mark conjunctions of the planets. I welcome Orion when he returns to the night sky. I feel graced by Venus as the morning star when she greets my dog and me in the dark mornings when we go out early for a walk. I hang imaginings on the hook of the crescent moon. At the full moon, I sing my longings to Luna's bright face. When I was teaching, I tried to encourage my students to recognize that, along with all the discoveries of what the earth has to offer, one of the great discoveries is to feel at home in the universe, to look into the starry firmament and feel that in this place you know you are known there for who you are. So it is not surprising that I found my way to offering something for a sense of well-being in this room where the planets and stars look down on the patient in the hospital bed.

Dr. Merryandrew: (Pointing to the mural on the wall near the bottom of the bed) Mylasia, do you see where we are?
Mylasia: In space?
Dr. Merryandrew: Right! On a spaceship in space. See, you can see the control panel of the spaceship in the corner here.

Mylasia: Oh yeah.

Dr. Merryandrew: Do you know any of those planets we can see out there in space?... What's that red one over there?

Mylasia: Umm… Mars?

Dr. Merryandrew: Yes, Mars. Do you recognize any others? What about the one with the rings around it?

Mylasia: Jupiter?

Dr. Merryandrew: That one is Saturn.

Mylasia: Oh yeah… I meant Saturn.

Mylasia is only ten years old. I would not expect her to know the names of the planets, but I always ask. Some younger children know them all and often older children do not recognize any. It seems to me that knowledge of the sky, like knowledge of the natural world on earth and the words that name dandelions, herons, otters, are vanishing from the education and experience of children. Regardless, I ask patients if they recognize any of the planets because it immediately engages them in the sky outside the window of the spaceship and we will be going into space together with imagination.

Dr. Merryandrew: What do you think that big white globe in space is?

Mylasia: The moon.

Dr. Merryandrew: Yeah, the moon. And what about that blue and green one?

Mylasia: That's earth.

Dr. Merryandrew: Great! The earth… Do you know that out there in space where we can see all the stars and planets, there is music? You know the earth and the moon and all the planets are spinning in space. And the earth is orbiting around the sun with all the planets. Even the sun and all the other stars are moving in space. As they are moving and spinning, they are making music. It's not the kind of music we listen to on the radio. It's not rock music, hiphop, jazz, country, gospel, or classical music. It's just beautiful tones that make up the kind of music we listen to on earth. The astronauts went out there in space and recorded that music with special instruments. At the Aerospace Museum in Washington, they play a recording of it.

I had been telling patients about the music in space without including the Aerospace Museum until one day a father sitting in a corner chair listening to me stopped me to say that what I was saying was true. He worked for awhile as a guard at the Aerospace Museum and used to hear the recorded music of space. I have not been up to the Aerospace Museum myself since I was a teenager, which was before space exploration, so I cannot corroborate what I was told that day. Though when I found out that gravitational waves were identified as sound, that seemed further corroboration. Anyway since it adds a note of authenticity, I have incorporated what I was told into my imagination of the music of space.

Dr. Merryandrew: They used to call that music in space the Music of the Spheres. Long ago, over two thousand and five hundred years ago, there was a guy named Pythagoras, who was a mathematician, who heard the Music of the Spheres. Two thousand and five hundred years ago the world didn't hum with motors and cars and electricity that buzzes in our ears. If you listen you can hear the fluorescent lights in this room buzzing. Back then there were no electric lights. The lights at night were fires and the stars. The world was a much quieter place than it is today. Pythagoras could go out in the night and see many more stars than we can see in places where there is artificial light. He could see the great river of stars we call the Milky Way and stars much farther away than that. He could also hear beautiful tones coming from the sky. The tones the planets made, he called those sounds the Music of the Spheres. In the Music of the Spheres, he identified the eight-tone scale of notes which is the scale used for most of the music we listen to today.

Obviously, Dr. Merryandrew takes an honest fool's license in spinning his tale. What he says about the eight-tone scale, or harmonic system, is not exactly accurate. Pythagoras is reputed to have discovered the intervals of the harmonic system by plucking strings of different lengths and listening for what sounds were pleasing and what sounds were not. He then noted the numeric ratios of the strings that made pleasing sounds. But for the sake of my sense of the wonder and mystery of music, I modify the story a bit.

When I was fourteen years old, I was introduced to Pythagoras by a book in my father's library called *The Magic of Numbers* by Eric Temple Bell. The argument of the book was that twentieth century science was changing after three centuries of grounding theory in experimentation to a return to the Pythagorean understanding that number rules the universe and the workings of the universe can best be understood by uniting theology and logic. In other words, the rules of the universe are not as apparent and observable as once thought. Regardless, for me as a young person what inspired me in reading about the Pythagoreans was their view that number had qualitative as well as quantitative value. We may all still recognize vestiges of Pythagorean thought when we consider the value we attribute to things that happen in threes or sevens. In my own mind, I have a Pythagorean view of music as manifesting the quantitative and qualitative values of number. A measure in music is a quantitative value that evokes a qualitative response. Consequently, I attribute to my early inspiration from Pythagoras how often what I do for patients includes song. For as Dr. Merryandrew attests, I sense in music some cosmic mystery of the balance and harmony needed for healing, which may well be quantitatively measurable and is most certainly qualitatively inspiring.

Dr. Merryandrew: We can't go up to Washington today to hear the recording of the Music of the Spheres in the Aerospace Museum. Nor do I think your mom is ready to have you travel into space to hear the music. So I'll tell you what I am going to do. I am going to download one of those beautiful tones from outer space into your room with an empty bowl and a magic wand. Don't I look like Harry Potter?

Mylasia: Uh… not exactly.

Dr. Merryandrew: OK, well maybe not… I know this stick doesn't look like a magic wand, but all I have to do is run the magic wand around the rim of the empty bowl like this and… Do you hear it? That's one of the beautiful tones from the Music of the Spheres. Listen. (Dr. Merryandrew plays the brass singing bowl and everyone in the room listens in silence.)

Mylasia: That's amazing. How do you do that?

Dr. Merryandrew: It's magic. (Still playing)

Mom: I'd like to listen to that as I go to sleep.

Dr. Merryandrew: It's hypnotizing… (Still playing… then stops playing) That's one of the beautiful tones from outer space, from the Music of the Spheres. There are other tones too. You know something interesting about the music of space, it's healing music. Because the music that is out there is in you, too. You know why? Because when the universe began – what some people call the Big Bang – in the beginning when light and dark were created and the stars and the galaxies, everything was set to beautiful tones of music. And we are all stardust. So we are all filled with music. Every organ of your body vibrates to a different tone, your heart, your stomach, your liver, every part of you vibrates to a different tone from the Music of the Spheres. If you listen for the music and you tune yourself to the music of the universe, you will be healthy… I've got a song about healing music. I'll sing you a little of it.

> *Don't play the drums that frighten the children*

Don't sing the songs about winning and
    losing
Sit down beside me the green fields are
    bleeding
Sing me the music of healing
Sing me a song of a lover returning
The darker the night the nearer the morning
Bring me the news of the new day that's
    dawning
Sing me the music of healing

Oh, oh the heart's a wonder
Stronger than the guns of thunder
Even when we're torn asunder
Love will come again

Somehow the cycle of vengeance keeps
    turning
Till each other sorrows and songs we start
    learning
Peace is the prize for those who are daring
Sing me the music of healing
Time is your friend it cures all your sorrows
But how can I wait till another tomorrow
One step today and a thousand will follow
Sing me the music of healing

Oh, oh the heart's a wonder
Stronger than the guns of thunder
Even when we're torn asunder
Love will come again[11]

These are the first and last verses of Irish singer song-writer Tommy Sands beautiful song, "The Music of Healing." Beginning with Pythagoras, who lived more than two thousand five hundred years ago, incorporating the ancient Tibetan singing bowl, and ending with a contemporary Irish song, this practice called the Harmonies of Healing seems to be Dr. Merryandrew's most culturally diverse imagination. Yet diverse as it is, no element is without justification for inclusion. Each has a legitimate contribution to make in the creation of a musical context meant to encourage a sense of well-being.

Although I said that Dr. Merryandrew takes a fool's license in his account of Pythagoras, in truth, he does not play as fast and free as it might seem. Maybe all that he expounds in regard to Pythagoras' capacities are not quit accepted fact. Yet in *The Golden Ratio: The Story of Phi, the World's Most Astonishing Number*, the author, Mario Livio reports:

The philosopher Porphyry (ca. A.D. 232 – 304), who wrote more than seventy works dealing with history, metaphysics, and literature, also wrote (as a part of his four-volume work *History of Philosophy*) a brief biography of Pythagoras: entitled *Life of Pythagoras*. In it, Porphyry says about Pythagoras: "He himself could hear the harmony of the Universe, and understood the music of the spheres, and the stars which move in concert with them, and which we cannot hear because of the limitations of our weak nature."[12]

So we can say that if not now, at least in another time more aware of soul capacities than our own, it was acknowledged that the great philosopher heard, listened to, and understood the music of the cosmos. And in that long ago time at the end of the Classical Period when Porphyry was writing, it was understood that only weakness prevented human beings from hearing what Pythagoras heard and feeling the sense of well-being that attunement to the harmonies in the cosmos can provide.

With regard to the singing bowl, initially, Dr. Merryandrew tucked the bowl into his magical

"Treasure Box" because I read in a book my wife gave me when she gave me the bowl many years ago, which book has now sadly gone astray, that the tone of the singing bowl has the power to close holes in "the etheric body." If I understand this notion correctly, the etheric body is the life force energy field around and penetrating into a living being. If there is a hole in the etheric body some of the life energy escapes, causing distress and illness. So the benefit of closing a hole in the etheric body would be understood as therapeutic healing. I mention this, however, not to suggest that this is my intention in playing the singing bowl. For in nothing I do in the hospital am I looking for medical results or evidence of physically measurable effects. In mentioning what I read about the effects of the singing bowl many years ago, I am only indicating that notions about the "etheric" may have been in the background of my thinking when I placed a singing bowl in Dr. Merryandrew's Treasure Box. Dr. Merryandrew plays the singing bowl with a simpler understanding that the tone the playing creates is soothing for anyone in the room – the patient, family members, nurses, techs and doctors. Like all sonorous music, the tone seems to penetrate into and envelop those who hear it.

As for Tommy Sands song, I think "The Music of Healing" recommends itself for use in a musical context dedicated to restoration of a sense of well-being even though it is not about physical illness. It is about social and psychological distress and as such makes its own claim for inclusion. It is one of the many songs in which Tommy Sands addresses the conflict in Northern Ireland. Yet even taken out of that context, it seems to make a universal assertion that healing music can overcome aggression, point toward the hope of a fresh new day, and re-form relationships with compassion and empathy. The song sings of the healing power of music to re-awaken relationships of love, as the refrain goes, "even when we're torn asunder/ love will come again."

Of course, none of the justifications for inclusion I have just given were in the forefront of Dr. Merryandrew's thought when this routine was being developed in service to patients. The comments on the Music of the Spheres, the playing of the singing bowl and the singing of "The Music of Healing" were brought together gradually over time during which experience, association and inspiration had equal parts in the creation. Yet in reflecting back over what came together in this routine, I recognize that the elements that were brought together are profoundly important as principles of establishing a sense of well-being as I understand it, namely, attune to the cosmos, sound a soothing tone, and relate with love.

Maybe it is no surprise that the fundamental principles of my work are revealed in a routine called the Harmonies of Healing, for in a sense everything I do in the hospital could be said to be practice to promote harmonies of healing. As I said at the beginning of this day of clown rounds, before entering a room, I tell myself to let go of my own thoughts and "Listen." I have asked the aesthetic question, is what I do well formed and worthy of the attention of others. I have asked the ethical question, do I bring some element of ease to patients, families, nurses and doctors, some ease in the context of dis-ease. And I have asked the spiritual questions about the meaningfulness of what I do. I have cocked a listening ear to the wind. In the wind, I hear a music of healing coming from the cosmos and at the bedside of patients. I have tried to shape what I do in accordance with the music I have heard. In everything I do I try to bring patients into relationship with the natural world which is our most intimate connection to the cosmos. And where I can I have tried to bring patients into relationship with the moon and the planets and the stars. In my lighthearted way, with a touch of levity, I have tried to establish a soothing tone in the buzzing busyness and frenzy of the hospital room. And I have met patients on their terms and served them to the best of my capacity with compassion and empathy.

At the end of *La Commedia*, in English known as *The Divine Comedy*, that is arguably the greatest poem of the Western Classical tradition, Dante recorded in the last Canto of the *Paradiso*, his final vision of a harmonious and unified universe. When he came face-to-face with the Triune Deity, he reports, he saw "how all the scattered leaves of the universe are bound by love in a single volume." (*Paradiso*, Canto XXXIII, ll. 85 – 87) I have read Dante's great poem many times over and taught it for many years. Knowing full well that Dante's medieval vision of unity and harmony in the cosmos was the last time in Western civilization that it has been understood that peace and stability reigned in the cosmos and recognizing that our contemporary vision is one of chaos and uncertainty, yet I have been inspired by the vision of the harmonious and unified universe that Dante presents. And in the work of Thomas Berry, whom I mentioned earlier, I have found the suggestion that we may yet return to a unified vision of the cosmos bound by a communion of subjects, that is to say, bound by love.

As a fool at work in a hospital, I cannot claim a stake in that great vision of unity that inspires me. And yet… and yet… in the stumbling way of a fool, I have found my way into a little glow of that greater light, accompanied by Pythagoras, a singing bowl and a fine Irish song. I have listened and I have heard a faint music coming from the cosmos and enveloping the bedside of patients. With my small portion of the greater vision, I uphold the hope of wholeness and unity, of a universe in which all the scattered leaves are bound by love. In the glow of that light, I sing the harmonies of healing.

Chapter Ten

Snagged in the Roots in the River of Life

Most of the time I do not get to see a patient for more than one hospital stay and whatever relationship can be established in the time of that one hospital visit is all the relationship there will be. That is as it should be. Unlike cardiology and pulmonary medicine, a positive aspect of pediatric medicine is that most of the patients do recover in a single hospital stay and do not return. Those with chronic disease, however, may return often. Children with asthma or sickle cell disease often return regularly. Face-to-face with what can seem like the monotonous drone of suffering that the need for frequent visits to the hospital creates, I try to have something new available to offer those patients I get to know over several years. Not that all those patients I see frequently always want something new from me. I have friends of many years who regularly request to talk with Jamie. But with those who want something to break the routine of a return visit to the hospital, I try to bring something new. With one boy with sickle cell disease who was often hospitalized for a pain crisis, over the years, I believe I sang every song in my repertoire, including the ones I learned when I heard he had arrived so that I could sing them to him the next day. And I try from time to time to update my storytelling repertoire.

I have known Taquisha for about five years or more. She is a child with sickle cell disease who seems to have had a number of pain crises each year over the years I have known her. Sometimes when I see her name on the days census, my heart sinks at the thought that she is suffering again. The disease is unrelenting, yet I never become inured to a child's frequent suffering. She is one who often requests long conversations with Jamie. Jamie, for his part, is always happy to greet her with his mix of love and sass.

Today, however, I promised her a story. I do not tell this story often because it is long and has a dark side to it that not just any older child is able to hear in the hospital. But since I have known Taquisha as she has grown up, I know she can handle it and it will take her out of the monotony of the hospital day for over an hour. Of course, I hope its merits are more than distraction; I hope it can offer her the entrancement of mystery.

Taquisha is a beautiful child with wide soft eyes that can melt your heart when she arrives at the hospital in pain. At those times she will just look sadly at you. If you ask her a question at those times, she only nods "yes" or "no." But when she starts to feel better, she smiles sweetly and talks quietly always giving you the sense that she is taking you into her confidence. Because of her gentle sensitive manner, I feel she is a good match for the heroine of the story I plan to tell her. Of course, like many sensitive people, she can be moody on any given day, especially if the effort to diminish the management of her pain sets her back. Hopefully that is not the case today.

Dr. Merryandrew: Good morning, almost afternoon, Taquisha. How are you doing?
Taquisha: I'm better. Maybe I'll go home tomorrow. How's Jamie?
Dr. Merryandrew: He's good. As much of a wise guy as ever. Right now he's chillin'. He wore himself out this morning. Luckily, I promised you a story. Maybe after I tell you my story, Jamie will have revived. Are you up for a story?
Taquisha: Is it a good story?
Dr. Merryandrew: Come on, do I tell bad stories? I wouldn't tell you a story I thought was bad. And

anyway I like this story. I think it's real good. It's a story that comes from Africa. I hope you like it.

One day when I was looking for a new story to tell, I read the original version of this story in Andrew Lang's *Lilac Fairy Book,* in which it is called "The One-handed Girl." I have stuck to the structure of the tale and adapted it, modified the language, added and eliminated parts of the tale, and generally changed it in ways that highlight different elements of the story and refocus it to emphasize parts of the tale that give it an entirely different feel. But it is still a variant of the Swahili story of "The One-handed Girl," which is a tale representative of a tale-type told in different versions around the world, probably the best known of which is the tale known as "The Handless Maiden" from the Grimm Brothers' collection.

Taquisha: OK, if you say it's good, I'm ready to hear it. Dr. Merryandrew: Good. As you know, Taquisha, as I have told you before, all my stories are old stories whether they are about things that happened long ago or things that happened yesterday. They are old stories because I learned from the old masters. The old masters knew that life is full of magic and miracle. They knew that there are spirits in the world who watch us even when we do not think that they are there. They knew that kindness and patience are as powerful as judgment and boldness for they invite a spirit to appear to heal a broken body, restore a broken life, and turn our hardships into gifts. Maybe if we listen to the old stories, we will know what the old masters knew. Maybe if more people hear the old stories, there will be more people around who know that life is full of magic and miracle.

In a land where food is often scarce and the jungles are full of danger, a girl and a boy lived on a small farm with their mother and father. They were only one year apart and were each other's only friend. All through their early years, brother and sister played together as their mother and father worked around the farm or traveled into the village. But as brother and sister grew up, they grew apart. The boy went off with the other boys of the village to play a ball game with a ball made of twisted and woven vines from the jungle. The girl stayed at home on the farm where she learned from her mother to cook and how to make healing medicine from the forest plants. In the village the boy met other boys who had wonderful things that he had never before seen. Sometimes he found something around the farm to trade for what the other boys had. And he began to feel his new things made him more like the other boys than like his sister.

When brother and sister were in their late teens, there was an epidemic throughout the land. Many people became ill and died. When their father contracted the illness, he called his children to him. He said to them both, "I do not know now how long I will live. I am not a wealthy man, but I have accumulated some few things that are in the house. I want you to choose. Will you have my blessing or my possessions?"

The boy answered, "I will have your possessions, father."

Then the father asked the girl the same question, "My daughter, will you have my blessing or my possessions?"

"I will have your blessing, father." Her father gave her his blessing.

In a few days, the father succumbed to the disease that had killed so many. Within the year after the father's death, the children's mother also became ill. She, too, called her children to her.

"I hear your father calling me, children. I will be leaving you soon, but before I leave you, you must choose whether you will have the possessions that are left or will you have my blessing."

The boy spoke first, "I will have the possessions, mother."

"And you my daughter?" The mother asked.

"I will have your blessing, mother." The mother

blessed her daughter. Soon after, the mother also succumbed to the disease.

With just the two of them left, the boy did not wish to stay on the farm. He told his sister that he would take what was coming to him. With those possessions he would become a traveling merchant. He would trade and sell things that people wanted in other villages and become a wealthy man like some who lived in their village. He left his sister only a small pot to cook in and a mortar to grind grain into flour. But there was no grain left in their home to grind. For when the mother had become ill, the family had used up all their small supply of food. The girl found only some pumpkin seeds on a shelf in the house. These she planted. But for the time being there was nothing to cook in the pot and the girl sat at home hungry.

Taquisha: She really got the bad part of the deal. Her brother should have left her something to trade for food. She didn't do anything to him. Why is he mean to her?

Dr. Merryandrew: Lucky for her things take a turn for the better.

As she sat wondering what she would do, a neighbor came to the house. The neighbor said her own pot had cracked in the fire when she was cooking and asked if she could borrow a pot to cook her meal in. She offered the girl some grain in exchange. So when the neighbor brought back the pot, the girl was able to cook a meal for herself. This happened again and again with other neighbors in the following days. It seems unusual that so many pots would crack in cooking fires. It makes me think the women of the village were looking out for her. But whatever the case, the girl was able to eat very well. And then one day, she went out to the field and found that a thick pumpkin vine was growing in the place where she planted the seeds. Pumpkins were already showing on the vine.

Time passed. News of his sister's easy life reached the brother, who had married when he made a little money trading. But soon after he had married, he had squandered all that he had. He envied his sister's good fortune and decided to go to see what he could get from her. He arrived before daybreak and saw sitting outside the house his sister's pot and mortar, which he had heard she loaned to the women of the village. He thought to himself, "These are the source of her good fortune. I will take them away with me. Then she will know hardship like mine."

Taquisha: Her brother is mean. What's his problem?

Dr. Merryandrew: At least she has the blessings of both her parents. Losing her pot and mortar doesn't turn out to be as bad as it seems.

When the girl awoke and went out in the morning, she discovered that the pot and the mortar had been stolen during the night. She could not imagine who would have stolen them since every woman in the village knew that they were hers. She did not know what she would do. But she determined to go to the field to see if her pumpkins were ripe. They were and there were so many that after she had enough for herself, she was able to take the rest to the village and exchange them for grain. Everyone who tasted the pumpkins said they were the sweetest they had ever had. Women came every day to trade for her pumpkins and soon she was able to buy herself a new pot and mortar.

The reputation of the pumpkins grew and one day her brother's wife came to buy pumpkins from the girl. It was late in the day and the girl was about to go home with the little she had left to make her own meal. When this stranger stopped her, she started to tell her there were no more, but when she learned it was her brother's wife, she gave her the largest pumpkin left and asked nothing in exchange.

The next day the brother's wife returned at the end of the day again to get a pumpkin from the girl. But this time the girl was returning home empty-handed and she told the woman there was nothing she could have.

When the brother heard this story from his wife, he thought that his sister had acted out of spite. He went the next day to confront her at her home.
Taquisha: Uh oh!!

Dr. Merryandrew: Her brother asked her why she had refused his wife. She told him, she had sold all her pumpkins and there would be no more pumpkins for awhile until the vine grew new ones.

"You are lying to me, sister. You are keeping them to sell to others. I will cut down your great pumpkin vine." His anger grew. He ran to where he knew the field to be. His sister followed. She knelt on the ground and put her hand on the vine to stop him from cutting it down and said, "If you cut down the vine, you will cut off my hand with it." But the brother was in a blind rage. He raised up his machete and brought it down, cutting off his sister's hand and the vine. Then without sympathy, he turned and left his sister bleeding where she was.
Taquisha: This is getting violent. Is this rated PG?
Dr. Merryandrew: Don't worry. You'll see. Hang in there with me.

When the girl could recover herself enough to stand, she went to the edge of the jungle and bound her arm in the healing leaves that her mother had instructed her to use. Then because she was afraid her brother would return to finish the job of killing her, she ran off into the jungle. There she wandered eating only what she found growing in the trees or on the ground and drinking water from the traveler's tree, named because it stores in the veins of its huge leaves quarts and quarts of potable water that thirsty travelers can find to drink. At night she climbed onto large limbs in trees where vines weaving through the branches could hide her from view and hold her in place when she fell asleep.

For a week she thought only of survival, but on the seventh morning in the forest, she woke with the recognition of all that had happened to her and she began to cry.

It happened that the son of a wealthy man with a great estate and land in many parts of the country had come very early on that day into the forest with a hunting party. But when they had been out for several hours, he grew tired as the sun rose and decided to rest under the shade of a tree. He asked his closest companion to stay with him and told the others to go on without him. There he fell asleep. He slept until he felt a drop on his face and woke thinking that it had started to rain. But when he opened his eyes, he saw the day was still bright. He put his finger on the wet place on his cheek and then put it on his tongue. It tasted of salt. Determined to find out where this was coming from, he climbed into the tree. There hidden behind vines on a high branch, he saw a beautiful woman crying.

"Are you a woman or a spirit of the tree?" he asked.

She stopped her tears and answered, "I am a woman."

"Why are you crying?"

"My troubles are too great to tell of in a tree," she answered him.

"Come back with me to my home. I will give you shelter and food to eat there. And you can tell me your story there."

"I cannot go with you. I am afraid for anyone to see me as I am," she said, holding up her wrapped hand.

"Don't worry. Wait here. I will send my friend away to join the rest of our hunting party. I alone will be with you and bring you to my home. If you wish, no one needs to know that you have come with me."

The young man climbed down to the ground and told his one companion to join the others of the hunting party. He told his friend that he had discovered a young woman in the tree who was greatly distressed. He was going to bring her to his house to see how he could help her. "But do not tell the others or anyone else about this."

When they were alone, the young man helped the woman down from the tree and together they went by the fastest route through the forest back to the young man's house, which was a small house on the property of his mother and father's estate. After a few days in which the girl recovered from wandering in the forest, the two young people found that they enjoyed being together. The young man went to his mother and father in the big house to tell them that he wished to marry and to ask their blessing.

"I have met a woman in the forest," he told them, "and I wish to marry her with your blessing."

They asked what he knew of her family and where she was from. But he told them that she had lost her family and her home and any place in the village from which she had come. He also told them about her hand. They wished that his heart had not gone to someone so unknown with only one hand. But he was their only son and they dearly loved him. So they gave the couple their blessing to be married. In time as they got to know their daughter-in-law, they came to love her too.

After a year, to their delight, a boy child was born to the young couple. Unfortunately, some months after the boy was born, the young man had to go to a far part of the country on business. He entrusted his young wife and child to his mother and father for safe keeping while he was away.

Coincidently, at the same time, the girl's brother, who believed his sister to have died, was traveling through the villages of the country. His wife had thrown him out for good and he had resumed the life of a traveling trader. He carried what he could on his back and traded in the open air markets of the villages where everything from food to wares was traded. In his travels, he came to the market of the village where his sister lived. There he overheard someone say to another, "Have you seen the wife of the son of the great lord of the village? I hear she has only one hand." When he heard this, he interrupted and asked, "Where did the lord's son meet this woman?" He was told, "Only one year ago, he brought her home from the forest." When he heard this, he recognized that his sister had again bettered her life, while his life had become more difficult; and envy ate at him.

Taquisha: Oh no, not the brother again!

Dr. Merryandrew: Yup, the brother again.

The next day the brother went to speak to the lord of the village. He spoke to the lord like the cunning trader he was.

"Sir, I have come with the intention to protect you. I have heard that you are kind and I fear that out of your kindness you have been deceived. Your son has married a woman with one hand. I know this woman. I shall tell you how she lost her hand. She is a witch. She married three husbands when she lived in my village and each one died because of her witchcraft. The people of our village discovered what had happened. They cut off her hand and sent her into the forest. If you do not get rid of her she will continue to murder, first your son, then others. Believe me and act before it is too late. I only come to protect you from this dangerous woman."

The lord believed what he heard because the trader spoke with confidence and cunning. The lord convinced his wife of the truth of what he was told. But they could not agree to have their daughter-in-law and grandson put to death as the stranger suggested even if she were a witch.

"We will do what her own village did and put her out in the forest."

They went to her and informed her that they knew that she was a witch and that they were going to have her and her son taken back to the forest where she could do no harm to anyone in their village or any other village.

With only an earthen cooking pot, mother and son were left in the forest. She wandered aimlessly wondering what she would do and how she would be able to care for her son. And when she grew tired she sat down at the roots of a tree to nurse her child to sleep. Suddenly a banded snake appeared nearby and approached them. Too frightened to move, she sat very still hoping the snake would pass them by. But when the snake reached them, it spoke.

"Open your pot and let me go in. Shelter me from the sun and I will shelter you from the rain."

She recognized that the snake had spoken a proverb of that country that she had heard many times before, "If you shelter your neighbor from the sun, your neighbor will shelter you from the rain." So she lifted the lid of the pot to let the snake climb in, then covered it again. Soon after she did the snake this courtesy, a mongoose came up to her. She knew that mongooses are the enemy of all snakes.

"Have you seen a snake pass this way?" asked the mongoose.

"Yes, it was moving very swiftly," she said.

"Then I will have to hurry to catch up." And off the mongoose went.

When the mongoose was out of sight, she lifted the lid of the pot and let the snake out.

"Thank you, for protecting me," he said. "Now tell me where you are going."

"I cannot tell you because I do not know. I was just wandering before I sat down here." And she told the snake how she had been put out in the forest with her child.

"Then we will go together to my home where you can find safety and rest," said the snake and he began to guide her through hidden trails through the thick jungle growth.

When they came to a river that is known in that country as "The River of Life" because its seasonal flooding irrigates the fields planted beside it and brings rich river bottom soil with the floods to renew the soil all around, the snake said, "We will rest here awhile. The sun of the day is hot and we have gone far. Take your baby and bathe in the place where the cool water of the river pools and the branches of the tree stretch over the water to shade the sun."

She waded into the water and as she bathed the baby with cool water, he splashed and laughed with delight. Then suddenly he arched and pushed with his legs against her at the same time and fell into the water and went under. She dived to pull him out but could not find him. She cried to the snake on the bank, "My boy is drowned."

Taquisha: This girl is cursed. Her parents must have said the wrong words when they blessed her.

Dr. Merryandrew: It does seem like that, doesn't it. Maybe this story should be called the girl of many sorrows. But... how could it be that she loses her son in a river called The River of Life. That seems wrong. And sure enough...

The snake called back, "Dive down again and feel everywhere. He may have become entwined in the roots of the tree."

She dived again, feeling everywhere with the fingers of her only hand. "No, he is not here. The river has taken him from me."

The snake called back again, "Dive again and search with both arms."

"I cannot. What is the use. I only have one hand," she cried. But she did what the snake told her to do. And her wounded arm touched something soft and round in

the roots of the tree. She lifted her son into the air. "My baby, my baby! He is alive. I have found him." The baby was happy and laughing and not at all frightened or hurt. She was so joyful, she hugged the child to her breast. And then she noticed that she had two hands; she had her lost hand back.
Taquisha: The snake knew that would happen, didn't he?
Dr. Merryandrew: I think you're right. He's not surprised when it happens.

"My hand! Snake, look I have grown my hand again," she cried and she burst into tears of joy.

"Now we must go quickly to my home, where I can repay you for the kindness you showed to me," said the snake.

"You have already given me so much. You have helped me rescue my baby and you have given me back my hand. What more could you give?"

The snake did not answer, but led again swiftly through the hidden trails in the thickets of the forest until they arrived at a hollow under the roots of a great tree where he lived with his mother and father. He told his family how he had escaped from the dreadful mongoose. When they heard his story, the mother and father were overwhelmed with gratitude. They insisted that the woman and boy stay with them and they would see to it that she and her child would be safe and provided what they needed. They gave her a room with a hammock in which to sleep and had their monkey friends bring fruit and coconuts filled with coconut milk from the trees so she and her son could eat and drink. She was content and at peace though she did not forget her husband.

Meanwhile her husband was away in the far part of the country for longer than expected because he had become ill while he was there and had to be nursed back to health before returning home. When many months later he returned home, he found that his father had hired a stranger to help on the land while he was away. The stranger had been a trader, but was happy to have the work on the estate and had done his best to make himself indispensible. Of course, the young lord asked immediately to see his wife and son. His father and mother told him, "She is dead."

"Dead?!" he cried out. "How could this be?"

Then he fell into great despair and for seven days he mourned. He took only water and did not come from his house. When he finally came from the house, no one dared to speak to him of his wife and child.

Who can tell if his wife, living in a tree in the forest among snakes, sensed his despair at such a great distance. They say that it can be that the communication between a couple can travel without sound or sight or by any other means. The message travels by magic. At any rate, one morning the woman told the snake, "You and your family have been very kind to me and I am at peace living with you. But I miss my husband and I wish that my boy could know his father. I would like to see if I might return to him."

The snake was sad when he heard this and said, "I will be grieved to see you go. You are loved here. There they put you out. But if you must go, first say farewell to my father and mother. And if they offer you a present, take nothing from them but my father's ring and my mother's small silver box."

She went to the father and mother to say farewell. They both had grown very attached to having her with them and wept at the thought of her leaving. They tried to persuade her to stay, but she would not. So they offered her gold and jewels as gifts with which to remember her stay with them. To their offers she refused.

"I shall never forget you, I assure you of that," she said. "If you wish to give me some tokens for remembrance, I will only accept your little ring and that small silver box. I will take nothing else."

The mother and father snakes did not expect such a request and had no desire to give these things away. These were the only things they did not offer to give. "Who told you to ask for these things?"

"Oh, no one," she said. "I only thought that because they are small, they would be easy to carry with me and I could have them for remembrance of my time with you."

"This is not true. We can tell that it was our son who told you to ask for these gifts. So it must be. Here is the ring. If you need food, or clothes, or a house, tell the ring and it will find you what you need," said the father.

"And here is the box," said the mother. "If you are unhappy or in danger, tell the box and it will comfort and protect you."

With the gifts, they gave her their blessings. The next morning, she took her son and left their home. She walked until she came near to the village where her husband and his mother and father lived. In a palm grove, she said to the ring she wanted a house. Immediately a house appeared in the grove. With her son in her arms, she went in the front door and at a table inside, she found food to eat. Because she had traveled a long way, she found that she was very hungry and ate immediately. After eating, she felt her fatigue and fell asleep with her son asleep at her side. She lived a quiet life there with no contact with the people of the village, but always hoping to be reunited with her husband one day.

Even though she had no contact outside her home and land, the people of the village wondered about the house that had gone up so quickly. They imagined fantastic stories about the woman who lived there. And those stories about the house in the palm grove reached the lord of the village. He wished to discover for himself who this woman was and if there were others living there who might threaten his family and the village. So with his son and the man he had hired to work on the land while his son was away, he planned to visit the house.

In the morning, the three men set out on the road to the house in the palms. The woman was outside with her son enjoying the cool air of the morning before the heat of the day. As she was playing with her boy on the ground in front of the house, a banded snake approached them. At first she was afraid for her son, but then she recognized her friend. He came close and told her how much he and his mother and father missed her and her boy.

"Many times, I have come by your house here to confirm that you are safe. That is why I have come this morning," he said. "I want to warn you that three men are coming along the road toward your house. I do not know if one is your husband. It may be that he is among them. But the oldest of the three is leading them."

"Thank you, my dear friend. I shall be careful in this meeting. If it is my husband and his father, I do not know who the third could be. I shall go inside with my son and prepare myself. I am grateful that you have come to me. How much I miss you and your mother and father and the monkeys who brought me fruits and milk."

"*You are always in our memory each day,*" *said the snake.*

"*And you in mine,*"*she said. Then she said goodbye to the snake and went inside with her son.*

When the three men arrived at her house, she met them at the door. She wore a veil over her head and face. She held her son by her side. As is the custom in that country, she invited them to come in, sit and share food with her before they spoke of why they had come. It was a wise custom for if guests arrived in anger, they would find it more difficult to express hostility when they had joined the hostess in a meal.

As they ate, the woman saw, indeed, that it was her husband and her father-in-law. And the third one was her brother. "Ah," she thought, "he must be the cause of my banishment. He must have spoken lies to my father-in-law while my husband was away. That must be why my father-in-law banished me to the forest." She saw that they did not recognize her. "How strange that these men, who know me so well, do not know who I am. Ah, of course, I have two hands. They cannot know."

"Now," said the father-in-law, "that we have been refreshed and well satisfied with your delicious food, tell us your story. There is much talk in the village about how quickly your house was built. During the time you have lived here, there has been too much talk about who the woman who lives in the palms must be. We hope you will

tell us who you are and where you have come from so we can reassure the people of the village. We can already tell them that you welcomed us with great hospitality and there is nothing for them to be afraid of."

The woman sat with her child beside her and began slowly to tell her story from the beginning. She saw that her brother became uneasy as she spoke. When the brother started to rise to run off, the older man made him sit back down. He sat frozen on his cushion beside the others, forced to hear all. When she reached the part of her story that recounted the meeting in the tree with her husband, her husband startled.

"It is my wife. It was a lie that I was told that you had died. And my boy is safe. This is my boy." He went to sit by her. "How could my father and mother have lied to me. But you cannot be my wife; you have two hands and my wife had only one."

"You must hear my story to the end." She told how her father-in-law accused her of being a witch and banished her to the forest. She told of the great adventure with the snake. She told about the boy snagged in the roots in The River of Life. She told how The River of Life gave her hand back. She told of the great kindness the snake family had shown her. But she did not reveal the powers of the ring and the box. She kept this secret to herself until a time when she could be alone with her husband. "These past months,

I have been waiting here in this house hoping to hear word of you and now you are here. We are restored to each other." So ended her story.

"My dear, what shall we do to this man, your brother, who has caused you such hardship all of your life?" asked her father-in-law.

Taquisha, what do you think they should do to him? Taquisha: Maybe they should cut off his hand. Or maybe they should cut out his tongue so he can't tell anymore lies to anyone. Isn't that the sort of thing that they did long ago?

Dr. Merryandrew: Yes, I think they did punish people with harsh punishments long ago. An eye for an eye. That was the sense of justice. But in this story it is different.

In that country, sentences in the courts of judgment were delivered with a proverb. The laws were meted out with words of wisdom. The brother knew this as well as anyone else. He heard for himself the words spoken to those convicted of crimes: "One cannot make a drum from a rotting log." This is how criminals were sentenced to death. He trembled as the words rang in his head. His sister spoke.

"It is true that my brother has caused me great hardship. And yet if I had not been forced into the forest from my village by his terrible act, I would not have met my husband. And if I had not been expelled

from your home, I would not have met the snake, nor would I have gotten my hand back. Perhaps it is right for him to be forgiven."

"Do you hear your sister's kindness?" the father-in-law asked the brother. "She is more generous than I would be if I were in her place. She has spoken kindly on your behalf. Yet your pardon must not be complete. You must have a place and time to learn the attitude of kindness that has never been a virtue in your life. Therefore you cannot stay within the village. As it is said, One cannot see the smoke inside a fog. One has to feel the heat and smell the burning to find the fire. As judge of the village, I send you from our midst to the dangers of the jungle that you learn the lesson you have missed."

With those words he sent the brother out. When the brother walked into the forest, the snake was watching. He knew what had happened in the house and he knew where the brother was headed. But for now, he just watched. He watched, too, as the father-in-law, the husband and wife and their child left the house to return to the great estate where they lived in peace and health for many years. When they had passed down the road and were out of sight, the snake watched as the house in the palms vanished.

Do we know who the snake was? No, no one can say for certain. But I have heard it said that he was one of the nature spirits who guide the lost, punish the unworthy and protect the innocent. He was one of the spirits who are always watching.

Taquisha: Wow! That was a good story. It started out a little scary, but that made the end feel really good. I didn't even want to get up to go to the bathroom... Don't leave while I use the bathroom.

Dr. Merryandrew: I'll wait. (Rita from food service arrives with Taquisha's lunch tray.) Hi, Rita. Taquisha just stepped into the bathroom for a minute. What's for lunch?

Rita: Good to see you, doctor. Taquisha ordered the chicken tenders and salad. And chocolate ice cream for dessert... How've you been?

Dr. Merryandrew: Life's been good, Lisa. How about you?

Rita: I can't complain.

Dr. Merryandrew: Well, that's not nothing... Oop, here's Taquisha... (As Taquisha gets back in bed)

You know what I always say about these old stories, Taquisha. You can put yourself somewhere in the story and it tells you something about where you are in your life. Are you deciding whether to choose material possessions or blessings in life? Are you making do with what you have? Are you crying about the hardships you've been through? Is there someone who makes you feel good about yourself even with all your flaws? Do you sometimes feel you are snagged in the roots in the river of life?

Taquisha: You've got to tell my sister that story when she comes in here sometime. (Taquisha's sister also has sickle cell disease.)

Rita: Here's your lunch, young lady. Did the doctor tell you a good story?

Taquisha: Yeah! It was a story from Africa. And it had a spirit snake in it.

Rita: Doctor, are you telling this girl scary stories about snakes? What are you trying to do, scare her out of the hospital?

Taquisha: It wasn't like that. The snake in the story is good. It's like the girl's guardian angel. The one who is scary is her brother. I'm glad I don't have a brother.

Rita: Well, I hope he didn't scare you away from boys. They're not all bad.

Dr. Merryandrew: Don't worry about that Rita. The girl in the story is rescued by a young wealthy lord and they get married.

Rita: Marrying into money sounds good to me.

Dr. Merryandrew: I'll try to remember to tell this story to your sister when she is here next time. Enjoy your lunch.

Taquisha: I will. Thank you.

Rita: I'll go out with you, doctor.

As I have said, I do not make it my business to interpret the stories I tell, but this story is a little different because it feels to me that the story itself is searching to get a handle on its meaning. At first it seems that like so many, this story has a certain inevitability to it. The bad seed brother is doomed; the sister is graced. Events in the story take shape accordingly as if the motivating force in the story is the course of destiny. Yet the one proverb mentioned in the story that might suggest an interpretation like that does not take hold. The brother thinks he will be sentenced with the words, "One cannot make a drum from a rotting log," but that is not spoken in his sentence. Instead he is sent out into the forest to learn from life experience and change and develop compassion. The words of his sentence are, "One cannot see the smoke inside a fog. One has to feel the heat and smell the burning to find the fire." Maybe the spirit of the snake will also be his guide, not as protector, but as the one who keeps his focus on what he must learn.

What it seems the brother needs to learn is what his sister has always known. He needs to get out of the fog of self-interest. He needs to learn, what we all have to learn, that the "fire" of life is kindled when one relates to others with empathy and compassion and love. He is sentenced to the forest as if to a primordial place of origin to learn the lesson of reciprocity as the foundation of empathy, compassion and love. That is the lesson spoken in a proverb early in the story by the snake: "If you shelter me from the sun, I will shelter you from the rain." Of course, as I said to Taquisha, what you find in the story depends on where you place yourself in it at any given moment of your life.

For me, the moment at the river captures the nearly inexpressible jolt that comes at the transition from suffering or illness to wholeness and a sense of well-being. Most of the time in the hospital, especially in Pediatrics, there is no sense of surprise or inspiration in the course of a patient's medical transition from disease to health. Doctors diagnose, treat and medicate, and chart the gradual process of healing. They ply their knowledge, science, skill and craftsmanship as they have been trained to do and as experience has taught them to do. But medicine is based on the statistical success rate and there are instances when things do not turn out as the statistics say they should. At such times, when concentration has been intensified by a problematic case or a near death experience, you can almost feel the jolt of transition when the patient is "out of the woods." You can almost hear it like the snap a broken bone makes when it is reset and goes back in place. I suspect that patients more often than those who treat them feel their turnarounds that take several days as bolts from a source of mystery. The return to wellness from illness can have that feeling if it is not subsumed under the rubrics of science. It is possible to recognize then that one can get snagged in the roots in the river of life and then magically be lifted up whole.

A few years into my work in the hospital, when I heard from a former student of mine whom I taught in high school, I tried to express something of what I feel about those magical moments when a patient returns to wellness after being snagged in the roots in the river of life. But I recognized in my letter to her how we can and most often do, overlook the magic and miracle of such moments and other important moments of transition in life. My former student was thanking me after many years for what I had taught her. She was, at the time she wrote, a medical student. I was moved to reply to her how much I admired her choice to be a doctor.

Dear C….,

It was lovely to hear from you. Thank you for your kind and generous words. I am moved that you credit me with affecting your life.

How wonderful that you are already beginning your rotations for your third year of medical school. I have been working in the hospital for over three years now and often I think, if I had it to do all over again, I would want to be a doctor. I would give up all my knowledge and understanding of the expressive life to be able to look back and say I saved one life. To think, five or ten years from now, you will be able to do just that. Maybe by then you will already know you have saved many lives. Of course, it won't seem heroic to you then. Maybe you will just think, "Looking back, I recognize that a few times I did the right thing at the right time for this or that patient. No more." But it will be enough. And you will recognize in your reflection your share in some other mystery, the Great Mystery.

I suppose as a teacher the best I can hope looking back is to say, "I, too, did the right thing at the right time and it made some kind of a difference in some students' lives." But it's harder to acknowledge as a teacher because it's never a matter of life and death. And I know I made my share of mistakes, too, along the way. I hope, however, as the Hippocratic Oath would have doctors forswear, I did no harm.

In my best moments, I think back and remember that I tried to hold a moral compass in my work. What I knew or thought I knew was that somehow I was preparing my students for that moment in each of their lives when they would have to confront evil face-to-face. I knew that the study of that confrontation was what *Faust* was all about and I set *Faust* as the final initiatory work we would all have to meet and try to understand in senior year.

But even though I taught *Faust* many times and have worried through the confrontation with evil all my life, I know I have not always met the challenge or temptation of evil with the good. Maybe because my reflections on the nature of evil began with study of extreme behavior and the criminal mind, in particular as evil was manifest in the Holocaust, I failed to recognize the ever-present influence of evil in daily life. My thinking has changed on that point. I suspect the great battle for good and evil plays out in each of our lives every day. Evil is not defined by object or agency; it is a relation. How we relate to the world and others we encounter during each day is as much as we can influence of our portion of the larger battle in which the moral universe is engaged. Often evil triumphs; sometimes not. It is not a question, certainly, of a quantitative balance sheet at the end. That much I have learned from Goethe's *Faust.* At best I think, it is a question of the grace that comes to us within our relations, as grace always comes, from a source unknown. How it comes is mystery, the Great Mystery. And yet though the gift of life and grace are both aspects of the Great Mystery, they are not the same and how they are different and integral in the Mystery is hard to say.

Miracle and mystery are still with us but we have grown autistic to the sound and form they take in everyday life. We don't notice the water has turned to wine, or maybe every now and then we do, but only when we turn and look quickly to the side. Nevertheless, ask any older doctor you can talk to about the Mystery and see what she (or he) says. Of course, don't ask bluntly like that; maybe ask about an unexplained cure or death she attended. If she doesn't have an answer, she's either lying or so stuck in medical ratiocination that she's forgotten. I know a young resident in pediatric medicine whom I am sure would have an answer for you. One day, I saw her crying in her office about a cancer patient we had lost in the unit. As you may have noticed, doctors don't usually cry, so she caught my attention. The few words she exchanged with me and her gesture when she came out of the office suggested to me that she was arguing with the Angel of Death, as if she had said something like, "OK, this time you got what you came for. But next time and the time after that and the time after that, I'll be more prepared. And in those encounters down the road, nothing is decided between you and me yet.

At the time I was writing, after three years in the hospital, I was well aware that in the routine of day-to-day life for a doctor or nurse as in the life of a teacher or many other forms of service work in the world, it is difficult to be conscious that at the heart of such work, most especially at the heart of medicine, there is an intimation of the miracle and mystery of life. Yet as an observant person privileged to work alongside those who are saving lives, I was in a position to be aware poignantly of what is at stake in the hospital, that patients enter the hospital snagged in the roots in the river of life and the heavy responsibility of those who treat them is to lift them up again through healing to wholeness. I was often in awe of what medicine can do. But I was also aware that sometimes mystery, the Great Mystery, breaks through the measured practices of medicine to impose a sense of humility and those in attendance have to recognize that some greater influence than their own has taken hold of the course of a life.

At the time, I felt I would like to have the skill and courage to practice an art that could bestow life. Working alongside those who practiced that art, I was questioning the meaning of what my art could do. I believed it mattered too, but how? I did not heal. As I have already said, I do not have the authority to assert a connection between positive emotional response and healing. To say that I just happened to do the right thing at the right time was not sufficient validation. Unlike teaching in which a teacher can see students' developing capacities to think and express themselves over time, what I offered patients would have to find validation in as little as one encounter. Obviously at the time, three years into the work, I had no answer. I believed what I was doing mattered. I held how it mattered as a question. I waited to live into an answer.

Chapter Eleven

La Commedia

I do not think I would have found my way to this work in the hospital if I had not had my own time snagged in the roots in the river of life. To be sure, many parts of my life experience converge in this work: four years of recording schoolchildren telling stories to each other for my dissertation for the Ph.D. in Folklore; thirty-five years of performing as a mime, actor and clown; the years I spent teaching ninth through twelfth grade humanities classes in the high school I helped found; a lifetime spent observing, learning about and appreciating the natural world; and the one time some years back, in her art gallery in New York City which she owns and directs, that my sister held a show of paintings to support the Clown Care program of the Big Apple Circus. Yet if I had not had a threatening hospital experience of my own, all those influences might never have landed me here. In my time in the hospital, I felt removed from all ordinary rhythms of my life. I felt submerged in a snarl of roots as the river of life flowed over me and away.

In my letter to my former student who was a third year medical student, I explained that I found myself a participant in the Great Mystery about which I was writing to her.

I once was the privileged recipient of a doctor's confrontation with death. I was dying in the hospital after my cancer operation. After my dire state had been described to me, a doctor from the same practice as my surgeon came into my room. I didn't know him. He spoke to the nurses with force and urgency. I could tell his adrenaline level was at battle pitch. Later I have thought, it was as if he had walked into my room and found the Angel of Death beside my bed. He squared off against the Angel and said without hesitation, "Get out! Get out!" and showed him the door. The rest of the story was good solid medicine. He ordered a chancy procedure. The head of radiological intervention performed the procedure perfectly. And a few days later,

I got to thank everyone for saving my life. I think the doctor who made the decision in my case remembers what happened that day in my room in something like the way I describe it. Why do I say that? Because he was not my doctor and should have let my doctor conduct the follow up visits after I left the hospital, but he insisted that he be the one to remove from my back the tubes that saved my life. The day he did that in his office was like a celebration of life. The man, whom I had seen in my room full of intensity and force, I discovered was light-hearted, easy-going and jovial by nature. Apparently he had prepared that celebration weeks before, because he told me that after he ordered the procedure that saved my life, he went back to his office and hacked into the radiology computer of the hospital to get the word on what was happening. As soon as he learned that the procedure was a success, there, alone in his office, he shouted out, "Yes," and shook his fist in the air in triumph. In that moment, I think he knew he had to finish out the celebration with me in his office. As you can hear, it was not just medicine as usual.

There is more to my story of my experience, of course, than I wrote in my letter to my former student in which my focus was primarily on those moments when a doctor finds himself at the threshold of mystery. In a fuller picture of my experience of being snagged in the roots in the river of life, I believe it will become apparent that it was there in my own experience as a patient in the hospital that my medical clowning had its origin and impetus. So this, I believe, is the appropriate moment to tell my own story. I do not tell it to be in any way self-serving. I am not like Coleridge's Ancient Mariner compelled to tell my tale. I am even now reluctant to do so. Yet I feel it is a significant part of the origin story of what I have said about being a medical clown and therefore belongs to the picture of the whole. For the sake of patient privacy, I have avoided saying much about the specific medical details for patients we have seen during this day. So perhaps my story can stand in for the experiences that I have had to leave out, not, to be sure, in its detail, rather in acknowledgement that the medical context of patients have been left out. For what looms large in my experience of patients, I recognize is a small part of patients' experience, but I hope not an insignificant part.

I was in my fifth year of teaching humanities at the high school I helped found when I was diagnosed with prostate cancer and scheduled for a robotically assisted prostatectomy. In the spring of the previous year, we had graduated the initial class that had started in ninth grade on the venture to create a high school at a school that had previously only gone to eighth grade. I had had the privilege to teach that class some of the great classic mythological works of the Western tradition: *Prometheus Bound,* Ovid's *Metamorphosis, The Odyssey, Parzival,* and *Faust.* I was scheduled after Thanksgiving of this fifth year of the school to teach Dante's *Divine Comedy* (titled simply *La Commedia* by Dante). My surgeon assured me that many who have the robotically assisted surgery go back to work in a week or two. But I decided to schedule my surgery for two days before Thanksgiving, give myself time to recover between Thanksgiving and Winter Break, which is notoriously a time when students are distracted by plans for the upcoming break anyway, and reschedule Dante for later in the early part of the new year. Little did my surgeon or I know that the journey of the pilgrim in *The Divine Comedy* down into Hell, up the mountain of Purgatory, and finally ascending into Paradise would have great relevance for my experience in the hospital or that Dante's great poem would be a theme running through the relationship between the surgeon and me till now these many years after the operation.

On the Monday of the week of Thanksgiving, I carried on as normally as possible. I took back the theater lights I had borrowed for the senior class play, which I had directed, and did the necessary preparation at home. By then I was confident that my health would be in the best of hands. My surgeon was well known as the best around. Nevertheless when I saw him earlier in the year, he had insisted that I discuss my options with a radiologist in the Cancer Center to get a second opinion. However, when I told the radiologist who had sent me to him, he bluntly stated, "If Dr. T___ is going to do your surgery, my advice is to go with it."

According to her account, on the day of surgery, my wife got concerned when my surgery went longer than expected, but she felt reassured by the doctor that everything went well. Within a day, however, first my kidneys failed to start up. Then when extra fluids got my kidneys functioning, my nurse discovered that I had a leak in the anastamosis because as fast as she emptied it, my Jackson-Pratt drain filled up again. As she alerted doctors of the problem, she attended to me with great equanimity, telling me stories of traveling to fairs with her father who was a potter whose pottery I had started to collect before he became renowned and had one of his pots brought to China as a state gift by the President. Even as doctors ordered different approaches to what was happening in my body, the nurse's storytelling kept me feeling that all would be well, all things would be well.

By the next morning, however, all was not well. I can give some measurable sense of the seriousness of my circumstances. Creatinine is a waste product of muscle processes that is ordinarily filtered out of the body by the kidneys. An acceptable range of creatinine in the blood is around 0.7mg/dl to 1.3mg/dl. My creatinine was at 5.9mg/dl. My weight had gone up from 125lbs to 152lbs overnight from fluid retention. A nephrologist came to see me early and told me there were three choices for me. Take me across town for dialysis, re-operate, or I was going to die. He delivered this message and then left. The male night nurse, whose shift was not yet over, came to see me when the doctor was gone. "Dave," I said to him. "I'm frightened."

This was an extraordinary moment. The nurse said nothing. He simply reached over and held my hand. If I had been drowning and he had perfectly tossed me a floating tube with a lifeline attached to it, that simple gesture could not have felt more reassuring. Of course, that was not the moment I knew I would live through it all, but it felt like a moment of grace. The three alternatives the nephrologist offered me all seemed to me to resolve in the third; the first two just more slowly. Yet the hand holding mine reassured me that someone would be with me and that was the reassurance I needed. He had spanned the space between us and joined with me where I was. That is what we mean when we speak of empathy and compassion, but that empathy without words was most powerful. I felt the tactile presence that told me someone was with me.

Soon after, as I described in my letter to my former student, the urologist from my doctor's practice arrived. He asked the nurse if they could attach the Jackson-Pratt drain to the wall suction. She warned him there was too much suction pressure for that. So he ordered nephritic tubes placed in my ureters in the hope that they would catch the urine headed to my bladder.

At this point in my morphine haze, I took the Gideon Bible from the drawer by the bed. Those were the days before the Bibles were removed from the hospitals. I turned to the Psalms and made sure I knew the 23rd Psalm by heart. When I closed the Bible I started to recite the psalm. The rest of the day, I believe I kept reciting it or, maybe because the morphine had slowed me down, it took me all day to recite it once as I left the room on my bed and waited in the hall outside radiology for the procedure.

When I was wheeled into the room and transferred to a prone position on the X-ray table, the radiologist squatted down to tell me what he was going to do. All I remember of that moment is that he had golden blonde hair and looked very young. In my haze, I did not understand that he was squatting; I thought he was very short. Just before I drifted off under the anesthesia, I thought to myself, "Great, a twelve year-old is going to do something to me."

A few days later when I asked to thank the radiologist for saving my life and he came to the room, I discovered to my surprise that he was about 6'8" tall. When I thanked him, he very humbly and matter-of-factly responded, "I'm glad it worked. It doesn't always."

The next day which was Thanksgiving, my surgeon, who was supposed to have the time off over the weekend, got himself up from the Thanksgiving table because he was worried and came to check on me. Although I was still heavily sedated on morphine, I was happy to see him. He has told me any number of times over the years since then that he felt I was a pleasant drunk, meaning that morphine did not make me hostile and angry. When he told me he was sorry that I was having to go through this, he tells me I responded, "It's not your fault. This is just typical of the way my body responds to any invasive procedure."

During the rest of the week that I had to stay in the hospital before going home, a wonderful Irish nurse tech sang me Irish songs as she took my vital signs and drew my blood. I also had the good fortune to have the same day nurse for the rest of the week. She would put her arm around me to support me as I walked down the hall each day, a little bit farther each day. As we made it along, she told me the saga of the vicissitudes of her married life, which kept my mind elsewhere than on my physical struggle to stay on my feet.

I left the hospital with four bags attached to four different drains in my body with the tremendous task for my wife of learning to measure my output each day and to redress the sterile bandages at my sites. A nurse told my wife she was getting a crash course in advanced nursing. When I was installed at home again, the homecare nurse, who checked on me several times during the two weeks I had all those tubes in me, looked at my chart on her first visit, looked up, and with a true New Yorker's irony that both tells the truth and makes light of it, said, "What are you doing here? From what I read here, you should be dead."

I have told my story with as much detail as I have, so that I could show how many moments of my stay in the hospital were taken up with expressive acts of others that saved me from self-absorption in my own predicament. There were the profound gesture of the night nurse who reached through the space between us simply to hold my hand; the stories of the nurse, the daughter of the potter, who told me about growing up with her dad as she emptied my drain; the marriage stories of the nurse who walked me down the hall each day; and the Irish songs of the nurse tech who took my vitals. Although I did not know it and would not have guessed, those gestures of others on my behalf became the foundation stones for my medical clowning four years later.

If I did not know then where my experience would lead or even if it would lead me anywhere, I did know I had been given a great gift by those who had attended me. In a letter of gratitude, I included a poem that expressed how privileged I felt I had been.

Cut from the web
   of my own life
      and falling
driven like a leaf
   un-limbed in the autumn wind
      or sinking
like a skipping stone
   that sinks
      when its final skip is done
I plunged in darkness
   toward a deeper darkness
      down
But I was held
   in a mesh of hands
      that caught me
strong and gentle
   old and young alike
      and when I woke
the web had been rewoven
   with threads and yarns
      of other human lives

And as the Advent season
    came upon us
        the story of the fall
had been rewritten as the story
    of new being by the many
        and the holy hands of grace

While I was convalescing at home during the holiday season, I tried to express in another poem my sense of the grace of being spared.

1

It is the evening of the festival of light
The umbrage of midwinter night
is over nature's calm and quiet of the
    storm withdrawn
The slow adagio of weather's symphony
played by the fingers of the ice-licked trees
now adumbrates in swelled tranquility
the near articulated mysteries
No fleet familiars in the cloudy sky
no starry swordsman moon and no great
    bear
disturb the awful sanctity of air
or pierce the atmosphere of pious prayer
with sudden pagan improprieties
It is the evening of the festival of light

2

Tu-whoo! A solitary visitor alights
upon a brittle shrouded bough to wait
for movement in the landscape of the
   snow
With round unblinking eyes that
   penetrate
the gloom he searches for the slightest
   sign
of weakness in the cold But nothing
   shows
No marking mars the purity of white
The sharpened beak and talons are
   resigned
Unsatisfied he glides behind the night
It is the evening of the festival of light

3

Now look within where phantoms of the
   firelight
cavort with shadows on the cottage wall
The flames convert substantial forms
to insubstantial silhouettes
and every object in the room acquires
   spectral life
as mist will rise from lake and stone
and consciousness from flesh and bone
Behold the simple cottager

asleep within his humble home
He dreams this night of wondrous birth
of transformations of the earth
of visitants and holy mirth
With intimations of the hour
he will awaken at the distant ring
of country bells to sounds of quiet
    murmurings
around the farm and choral harmonies
descending from the mountain heights

4

It is the evening of the festival of light
The umbrage of midwinter night
is over nature's calm and quiet of the
    storm withdrawn
The slow adagio of weather's symphony
played by the fingers of the ice-licked
    trees
now adumbrates in swelled tranquility
the near articulated mysteries
No fleet familiars in the cloudy sky
no starry swordsman moon and no great
    bear
disturb the awful sanctity of air
or pierce the atmosphere of pious prayer
with sudden pagan improprieties

I taught my postponed Dante class at the rescheduled time in February. Yet curiously though not in a disturbing way, Dante has continued to haunt me through the years. Eight years after my operation, I gave a series of seminars on Dante's *Divine Comedy* and the work of Thomas Berry. I published a little book from the seminars entitled, *All the Scattered Leaves of the Universe: Journey and Vision in Dante's Divine Comedy and the Work of Thomas Berry.* On New Year's Eve that year, I happened to be bringing a copy of a talk I gave about that book to Thomas Berry's sister, Margaret, who had supported me in the work I had done for the book. When I handed her the envelope with the text of the talk, Margaret asked me how I had become such an expert on Dante. Since she had taught Dante for more years than I had (forty or fifty years, I believe), I felt that I was safe in responding that she herself would understand how when you teach something for awhile you start to think you know something about it. What I did not say to her, however, was that, although I do not consider myself an expert by any means, I had once lingered in a liminal realm that had given me some special insight into Dante's vision.

Recently in this year of the Covid pandemic when I went to see my surgeon for my annual checkup, Dr. T____ told me he was rereading Dante. "When this pandemic is over," he said, "we'll have to go to lunch together so I can pick your brain about Dante." He also told me that of the hundreds of robotically-assisted prostatectomies he has done, I am the only patient he has ever had who needed nephritic tubes. Like I said years ago, "Doc, it's not your fault; it's just me." The fate of a fool.

I figure my work in the hospital is in part a gift to me from my tribulations at the time of my surgery. And in the spirit of reciprocity, my work as a medical clown is in part a gift of gratitude returned in response to the gift I was given.

Chapter Twelve

The Fool in Community

When I first came to the hospital, I thought that it would be much as it had been for me in the thirty-five years I spent traveling as a solo mime/clown. I would come to the hospital, perform my clown rounds and leave. I expected that I would be recognized, but otherwise unnoticed and unacknowledged by those who had a more permanent place than mine in the hospital setting or even by families and patients whose rooms were not on my census to visit. When I was a traveling performer for all those years, even when I had a stretch of a week or two as an artist-in-residence in a school and was provided lodging by a teacher or a family of a student in the school, I never gained status in the community as anything more than a guest. I suspected that I would be regarded in the same way in the hospital as I had been regarded in my years of traveling, which is to say as an outsider.

I imagined that as an individual I would move through the interstices of the medical world of the hospital without ever becoming a part of it. Dr. Merryandrew expected to serve patients in the best way he could and to build a repertoire of options for things to do when entering a room. When part of my work became encouraging everyone in the room to join in interaction surrounding the patient, I felt the little community that formed in the room was hardly more than an ephemeral creation. For I had no other expectation than that as Dr. Merryandrew left, patients, family members, friends, nurses and doctors would revert to the isolated spheres of their lives, patients to their suffering or distractions on their devices; parents to their cellphones or computers; nurses to their tasks of setting and adjusting IVs and entering data in patient charts; doctors to their diagnoses and attention to others. The little community in the room would likely evaporate as Dr. Merryandrew withdrew. Yet to my surprise and despite my expectations, Dr. Merryandrew's effect seemed to endure, at least in some ways. For Dr. Merryandrew became a recognized figure in different tiers of the hospital community and an acknowledged member of the hospital's multi-tiered community.

After a few months as a presence in Pediatrics, I became a recognized service of the unit. Though it was very rare for medical staff to ask me to help in a room, patients and families did occasionally ask for me and many more expected me to knock on the door as I made my rounds and welcomed me when I did. And attending physicians with the pharmacist, psychologist, and social worker, all making rounds with the team of residents and medical students deferred to me if they found me in their next room and re-routed to give me time with the patient.

Around the hospital halls outside the unit, I became familiar with members of the staff and as one friend generously labeled me, I became a "fellow co-worker." Days begin by touching base with staff and volunteers at the information desk at the entrance to the hospital. Sometimes I have sung a song there or Jamie has made a surprise visit. Sometimes I am stopped right there at the desk by someone who requests that I come to the room of a family member in a unit other than Pediatrics and I am always happy to oblige the request.

One encounter in the hall is noteworthy for the poignancy of the synchronicity of the moment. I was entering the hospital for the day when a man coming down the hall caught my eye. I noticed him because he looked like he had just come into the hospital from a farm. At least I was certain he lived out in the country away from town. I expected him to take no notice of me as he passed by and out the door. But as we approached each other in the hall, he came up to me, which surprised me. To add to my surprise, he asked where he could get a nose like mine. He said his sister was dying in the hospital and he wanted to brighten up her day a little. I looked at him with a sense of astonishment at that point. The two of us, who seemed to have no life experience in common, actually had more in common than ever could be guessed. Several hundred miles away in Cambridge, Massachusetts, my own sister was also dying. Moreover, for some unexplained reason, the day before, I had bought a brand new cellophane wrapped clip-on clown nose at Walgreens and put it into my Treasure Box just on the chance I might have a use for it, or as my sister would put it, "just in case." There we were, two brothers who shared concern for our sisters who were dying. Of course, I gave him the clown nose in my chest. And so we passed in and out of each other's life.

To my surprise then, I have become a distinguishably unique figure in the multi-tiered hospital community. That has set me to reflecting on my role here. I do so recognizing that however long I have been here, there will always be those at every tier of the community who do not accept the presence of a clown in their midst.

In my reflections, I have come to realize that just as a doctor in the hospital represents for others the archetype of Healer, as a clown in the hospital, I too present an archetypal image to others. That archetype is not the archetype of the Healer though I wear the doctor's lab coat. As I have said, I claim no expertise to assess whether or not the emotional shift I try to affect in patients has any measurable medical outcome. The image I present is the comic archetype of the Clown/Trickster/Fool. I am aware that the terms "clown," "trickster" and "fool" have acquired many different connotations in our cultural context and may evoke connotations I do not intend. So I will need to define what I mean when I say that I present the archetype of the Clown/Trickster/Fool.

The place I want to begin is with a very simple definition of the comic spirit. It is a definition I always used with my ninth grade students in our seminar on Comedy and Tragedy. I came across this definition of the spirit of comedy in the wonderful book, *Telling the Truth: The Gospel as Tragedy, Comedy and Fairy Tale* by Frederick Buechner.

> The comic is the unforeseeable. How can Donald Duck foresee that after being run over by a steamroller he will pick himself up on the other side as flat as a pancake for a few seconds but alive and squawking? How can Charlie Chaplin in his baggy pants and derby hat foresee that though he is stood up by the girl and clobbered over the head by the policeman and hit in the kisser with a custard pie, he will emerge dapper and gallant to the end, twirling his invincible cane and twitching his invincible moustache?[13]

Not only is the comic defined by the unforeseeable as Buechner says; the comic is also, as Buechner distinguishes it, that spirit in life that carries with it the gift for recovery. Donald Duck is run over and still returns to life. Whatever misfortune he suffers, Charlie walks away from it as gallant and invincible as ever. Donald and Charlie are figures on the road that keeps on going, emblems of the eternal journey of life and the spirit that sustains us through all our vicissitudes.

This is the vision of life to which King Lear poignantly appeals at the end of Shakespeare's great tragedy. Though Cordelia declares to him that they have incurred the worst that the world can give, he says too late to the only daughter who has ever loved him: "Come, let's away to prison:/ We two alone will sing like birds i' the cage:/…so we'll live,/And pray, and sing, and tell old tales, and laugh/… And take upon 's the mystery of things…" (V, iii, 9-10,12-13,17) Lear's words and the vision of life they express echo for me through so much of what I do. In the midst of unceasing tragedy, they give voice to the comic spirit and vision. When I say that Dr. Merryandrew seems to present others with an image of the comic archetype of the Clown/Trickster/Fool, I am suggesting that as a clown doctor he evokes that spirit deep within that we share with all humanity by which we shrug off our hardships and go onward into life to sing and tell old tales and laugh again.

A priest I often encounter in the hospital has repeated to me any number of times that he and I are in the same business. I never disagree with him, but I do consider there to be a great difference between the kind of grace we bring to the bedside of patients. With his clerical collar, prayers, and Holy Book, my friend offers the grace of transcendence to his parishioners. He offers the grace that lifts their souls above their human dust into the realm of pure spirit. I cannot offer that. The Clown/Trickster/Fool embodies the naturalistic vision of the indomitable spirit of life that picks us up when we fall and though we are still soiled with the grime of the fall, that spirit sets us back on the road to our journeys destination. If there is grace in that, the grace it offers is no more, yet also no less, than the immanent grace that inheres in a handful of stardust.

A good part of my understanding of what it means to enact the archetype of Clown/Trickster/Fool comes from a perspective that has nothing at all to do with comedy. It is a perspective that Dr. Rachel Naomi Remen writes about in her beautiful book, *My Grandfather's Blessings: Stories of Strength, Refuge and Belonging.* In her introduction to the book, Dr. Remen writes about her experience of her grandfather, who was a rabbi and a scholar of Kabbalah, the mystical teachings of Judaism. From him she learned of a vision of creation in which light was poured into the vessels intended to receive the creation, but the emanation proved too powerful. The vessels broke and shattered, scattering shards of light throughout the universe.

From this vision, Dr. Remen observes:

> There is a god spark in everyone and
> in everything, a sort of diaspora of
> goodness. God's immanent presence
> among us is encountered daily in the
> most simple, humble and ordinary ways.
> The Kabbalah teaches that the Holy may
> speak to you from its many hidden places
> at any time. The world may whisper in
> your ear or the spark of God in you may
> whisper in your heart. My grandfather
> showed me how to listen.[14]

In the vision of the shattering of the vessels,
the Kabbalah said that the purpose of a life of
service was to gather up as many of the shards
of light as possible to restore the universe to the
wholeness of its origin. Throughout her life, Dr.
Remen has pursued this sense of service and she
writes about her experience:

> As a young doctor, I thought that
> serving life was a thing of drama and
> action and split-second judgment calls. A
> question of going sleepless and riding in
> ambulances and outwitting the angel of

death. A role open only to those who have prepared themselves for years. Service was larger than ordinary life, and those who served were larger than life also. But I know now that this is only the least part of the nature of service. That service is small and quiet and everywhere. That far more often we serve by who we are and not what we know. And everyone serves whether they know it or not.[15]

Again Dr. Remen's grandfather told her of the nature of true service by teaching her the legend of the Lamed-Vovs. The story tells that God will allow the world to continue as long as there is a minimum of thirty-six good people in the world who are capable of responding to suffering. These thirty-six are called the Lamed-Vovs or Lamed-Vovniks. If there are fewer than thirty-six such people, the world will come to an end. He told her since no one knows who these thirty-six are, anyone you meet might be one of the thirty-six. Her grandfather said, "It is important to treat everyone as if this might be so." When she heard this story as a child, Dr. Remen reports she puzzled about it and asked her grandfather to explain. She writes that as a child, she understood that people were supposed to do something in return for the gift of life, but she did not know what.

> Suddenly, I realized that I had no idea what it was. If so much depended on it, it must be something very hard, something that required a great sacrifice. What if the Lamed-Vovniks could not do it? What then? "How do the Lamed-Vovniks respond to the suffering, Grandpa?" I asked, suddenly anxious. "What do they have to do?" My grandfather smiled at me very tenderly... "They do not need to do anything. They respond to all suffering with compassion. Without compassion, the world cannot continue. Our compassion blesses and sustains the world."[16]

Dr. Remen's vision of light and life and listening sustains me in my work and stands behind my understanding of the archetypal role I play.

My friend the priest, at times, comes to the hospital to attend at the bedside of the dying. Even with my much more limited experience with adult patients, I have also been asked to come to the bedside of patients who are terminally ill. I have asked myself as others might ask, is it appropriate for me in my clown nose and pork pie hat to enter the room of a patient who is terminally ill. Of course, I am there because a family member has requested that I come, but I am sure there are those who would question with me, do I belong. Over time I have come to answer myself, and those who might ask, that, yes, I do belong as representative of the comic archetype in the context of dying. I have the greatest respect for my clerical friend who promises transcendence for the dying. I honor the gift of that grace. Although I have never discussed it with him, however, I believe he would say that I belong there too. For if he offers the gift of what comes from the realm beyond this life, I offer affirmation of the life as lived, life as the rugged journey we all must live made up of our little triumphs and the failures we have passed through and overcome, of our successes and mistakes and the place to which life has taken us. I enter the room to honor and respect that somewhere for the patient in the room, if one listens, one will hear the music of the spheres that inheres in the body and sense the light that exalts the soul. Somewhere in the dying embers, the spark of creation still burns.

I know that when I invoke an archetype, I refer to the symbolic figures Carl Jung identified as residing in the depth of the collective unconscious that we share with all humanity and to which anyone has access. There is really nothing grandiose about this. Archetypes are our common heritage. In invoking an archetype, I am trying to bring understanding to the role that I play in the lives of the patients I see and in the community of the hospital. In another sense, too, I am trying to recognize and understand the responsibility I have as a figure in the lives of patients, a figure who, more than a personality, represents a universal type. And I must add that an important part of becoming aware of the function of the archetype includes recognizing that it was Jung's understanding that every archetype possesses within itself the seed of its opposite.

Take for example, what I identified as the doctor's archetype, the archetype of the Healer. In her personal and inspiring book, entitled *Slow Medicine: The Way of Healing*, Victoria Sweet identifies what she refers to as the archetype of the Physician with the Jungian archetype of the Wise Old Man. She writes in a note regarding her use of the notion of the archetype of the Physician.

> Jung touches upon the most important
> aspect of this archetype, I believe, when

he emphasizes that the Wise Old Man is "a life-bringer as well as a death-dealer… Indeed the old man has a wicked aspect too, much as the primitive medicine-man is a healer and helper and also the dreaded concocter of poisons." The ambiguous aspect of this archetype that the doctor plays into is why there is so much expected of us – the virtues of mother, father, saint. He who can cure can also cause; he who can heal can also afflict; he who can save a life can also take a life. So the archetype of the Doctor is the archetype of the Magician.[17]

I believe that what she says about the ambiguity of the archetype of the Doctor affects those who have what is known as "white-coat syndrome." It is well-known that there are people who will not go to a doctor because as my own grandfather used to say, "Doctors are the only people licensed to kill you." My grandfather said this despite the fact that he made such a great contribution to the building of North Shore Hospital on Long Island that a wing of the hospital is named after him.

Similarly the archetype of the Clown/Trickster/Fool possesses an ambiguity. It represents the comic spirit of affirmation, of life eternally renewing itself in the face of adversity, and at the same time contains within it the seed of what undoes our lives. Trickster creates the world and dismantles it. I am well aware that my own presence in the hospital as Dr. Merryandrew can inspire such ambiguity. As I mentioned at the beginning of this day, I recognize that there are those who assume only the negative when they see a clown in the hospital. They sometimes mention to me some negative image or experience they once had with a clown. I cannot argue with that and do not try. I accept that they do not wish to see me and I do not impose. I modestly hope that in stepping away graciously I leave behind the residue of a positive gesture of acceptance of how they feel that may weigh against the negativity.

In truth, I myself have certain idiosyncratic associations with the ambiguity of the archetype that I enact. As it happened when I began at the hospital, I bought myself two lab coats at the local scrubs store. Since I am between sizes, I bought one in a smaller size and one in a larger size; one is a little tight, one is more roomy. But I did not think the differences in sizes would matter very much, and they do not really, except for what I discovered to be my own associations with the difference.

My association with the smaller coat can be explained very simply. The short sleeves, the tightness at the shoulders feels Chaplinesque. Charlie Chaplin's famous character of the Little Tramp with his moustache, cane and bowler hat wore a jacket that was too small for him. Since I have already said that Chaplin is my model of the enduring comic spirit, it is no surprise that I might make this association. It is, to be sure, a positive association.

My association with the larger coat is more obscure. During World War II when France was under the Vichy government, a classic Romantic movie was made in the south of France. The title of the film was *Les Enfants du Paradis* (*Children of Paradise*). It tells the story of Jean Baptiste Gaspard Debureau, a performer in the Theatre des Funambules, the pantomime theater situated in the Boulevard of Crime in Paris in the 1840s. Debureau took on the minor character of Pierrot in performances. When he started to perform, Pierrot as a character was little more than an expression of ennui. Debureau, however, transformed the character into a romantic dreamer and the expression of the sensitive aesthetic soul. He captured the imagination of poets and artists and made the obscure theater in the Boulevard of

Crime into a sensational attraction for the theater goers of Paris. In the film, Debureau was played by Jean-Louis Barrault who would become one of France's greatest performers and directors. At the time of the movie, with Etienne Decroux, who would become the teacher of several generations of mimes including Marcel Marceau, Barrault had already developed a new French physical theater which would spawn the style of twentieth century illusionary mime. Decroux was also in the movie and played the part of Anselme Debureau, the father of Baptiste. Without going into the story, I think I have said enough to indicate that the story of the film and the performers in it represent the heritage I acquired when I became a mime. My own professional lineage is directly joined to that heritage since one of my teachers was Marcel Marceau. For many mimes in the latter half of the Twentieth Century, including me, *Les Enfants du Paradis* was the inspiration for our choice of career. The impression the film made on me and the mystique surrounding it created by the stories about its making during dark days under the Vichy government has never left me.

It is with a character in *Les Enfants du Paradis* that I make an association with my larger lab coat. There is a minor character in the film named

Jericho, who is identified as an old clothes man. Jericho weaves through the various plot threads of the story peddling old clothes, books, and fortunes as a representative of the seamy side of the Boulevard of Crime. I can give a couple examples of how he introduces himself into a scene as a way of giving a sense of his character. In one scene in a tavern, he is brandishing an almanac in the air and speaks in a drunken voice.

> "Have you been dreaming of cats? Have you been dreaming of dogs? Have you been dreaming of troubled waters? Here is the explanation of all your dreams…"[18]

In another scene, this time backstage at the Funambules, he introduces himself as a meddler in other people's affairs.

> "Here's old Jericho, known as the Wild Boar, known as the One who Sleeps by Himself!... I've always lived alone, so, of course, I interest myself in other people… it's only natural… Always alone, that's no life! Nobody ever loved me, nobody, zero, nothing! even if I was a widower, at least I'd have some memories…"[19]

Jericho's peddler's costume looks much like that of a tramp clown with crushed top hat and ragged baggy jacket that seems too loose on him. There is, however, nothing humorous about his character. His impact is powerfully negative and disturbs Baptiste every time he appears. It is almost as if in this one character the writer, Jacques Prevert, himself a poet, found a way to express the desolation of his war-torn country during World War II and the bitterness, desperation and defeat many felt at the time. And for me, Jericho and the mood he creates around him constitute my image of the clown turned negative.

Sometimes when I am wearing my lab coat that is slightly too big, I recall the somber, frightening image of Jericho and worry about the image I present. I am visited by the dark side of the archetype. I never let it linger with me. The next day I will change my lab coat to release the negative association though I do not let either of my associations play into what I do. For I do not see myself as Chaplinesque, or as evoking in others the mood of Jericho. But my associations make me ponder an ambiguity that is there.

So when people in any tier of the community of the hospital reject my presence, I am not offended. In fact, I accept that with their rejection they are registering that I have evoked for them the dark side of the archetype of the Clown/Trickster/Fool. I am grateful, however, that the majority feel the lightness of my presence.

It may seem, beside the productivity and business of the hospital, that these considerations regarding the archetype of Clown/Trickster/Fool are trivial. Yet I believe to bring any such images into the focus of conscious awareness exposes the figures and colors that play across the canvas of our lives. And the awareness adds enchantment to our days. Awareness also makes it possible to avoid playing into the negative influences of the psyche. Every day I walk into the hospital, I am aware that I activate an archetype from the ancient store in the collective unconscious of humanity. As I walk through the hospital halls, I awaken to awareness of the significance of the role that I play in the lives of the community. I accept that the role of the clown comes with responsibility. I try to deflect the negativity that inheres in the archetype and to honor the spirit within each one of us that brings a smile to the face at the end of a hard day, helps us scramble up when we have fallen, brings a light to the eyes, a song to the heart and the promise of recovery when someone we know and care for falls ill.

Chapter Thirteen

Listening with Softened Eyes

There is a Native American instruction for one entering the woods that I used to recommend to my high school students when I wanted them to be present and reverent as I took them out into the forest beside our school to write poetry or reflect on the Transcendentalism of Emerson and Thoreau. The instruction given was to "soften the eyes." To understand what it means to "soften the eyes," let me first consider its more common opposite, what it means to have hard eyes.

We live in a culture that is dominated by the sense of sight. Most of the time we focus our sight. We look out at the world around us every day without a sense of our integral place within it. We read, we look at screens, we watch sports events and celebrations, all with focused sight. We see the world and others as objects of attention. Focused sight is hard sight; it fixes on the object of attention. And what we perceive is most often filtered by what we already know about an object or another. We see what we are prepared to see.

When we soften the eyes, our gaze becomes diffused. We expand our field of vision and see everything in relation to everything else. In this diffused way of seeing we let go of what we know, we let go of the chattering of the I behind the eye, and bring ourselves into presence with the world and others with a sense of deep relation and connection. We recognize ourselves as subjects among subjects. As Thomas Berry said, the world becomes "a communion of subjects, not a collection of objects."

Earlier, I mentioned what I listen for in my work as a medical clown. I carry aesthetic, ethical and spiritual questions as I work and listen. I initially started out listening with attention and questions focused on aesthetic, ethical and spiritual considerations. With time my listening has become less focused, more diffused. When I stand at the door to a room preparing to listen, I remind myself to release what I know, let go of what I have brought with me, soften my eyes to recognize the connections in the room and be present to the patient before me, surrender to the moment. I call this "listening with softened eyes" because I am listening as a subject among subjects.

In describing listening this way, I do not confuse being present to another with the emotional responses of sympathy and antipathy. For being present does not involve an introspective turn. "Listening with softened eyes" is like standing at the end of a dock at night and looking up at the stars in the dark sky overhead, feeling the wind coming in off the sea, smelling and tasting the salt in the air and hearing the lapping of the waves in at the shore. At such a moment one is overwhelmed with reverence. The gaze is turned outward. The mind has stilled its impetuous activity. The ear beholds the thin silence at the heart of things and the fullness of it.

In introducing my work, I broadened the definition of health to incorporate the status of the soul and the soul's capacity to engage with another and with the mystery of life. As I said, with this broader definition, I recognized that health can be measured with laughter, as well as with seriousness. It can be met with a light heart, as well as solemnity. There is in it a quality that cannot be quantified, but we can know it and sense it in ourselves and recognize it in others as a positive state of well-being. Absence of pain or infection is not the only measure of health; health is also encountered and expressed in a sense of beauty, a sense of humor, appreciation of music and song, as alignment with the animal and vegetable kingdoms of nature, as the capacity to imagine, as ability and willingness to be drawn into the tensions of a story, and, of course, as acknowledgement and response to another. I called this broader sense of health a sense of well-being. As I entered into the work, I hoped to promote a sense of well-being with my tales and folly. I have found that to do that I needed to listen with softened eyes.

Looking back over the years, I see how much what I have done defines and explores hospitalization as liminal. In a place isolated from the traffic of life, time stands still in the rush of our days. Yet the feeling of isolation in place and of being arrested in time is only part of what defines hospitalization as liminal. More profoundly, I have come to recognize that hospitalization is experienced and to be understood as a transitional and transformational moment in life. It is as transitional and transformational experience that hospitalization is most profoundly to be identified as liminal. This is a very different way of looking at illness than the ordinary view of illness as an experience to be overcome and hospitalization as a time to get fixed when the body is broken or diseased. I recognize that most of what I thought I was developing as isolated routines and stories were discoveries made to help patients see their hospitalization as a time for transformation and to help them make the transitions to which this moment in their lives had brought them.

When I was hospitalized, I found myself to be in a liminal reality. I was snagged in the roots in the river of life in an eddy of time. In my confusion and uncertainty, I sensed myself and the moment as empty and full like a place and time of both dissolution and creation where some things were ending and others were coming to be. Unable to do anything for myself, I accepted what others brought me as gifts – their medical expertise, their simple human presence and touch, their stories and songs. And I was lifted and raised by them, changed yet whole again. In these past years, with a sense of what was done for me, I have tried to find ways of my own to serve others as I was served. So much of what I have found pertains to my sense of the liminal reality I found myself in as a patient. And I have come to appreciate ever more deeply, than I did even then, that liminal reality is a time when life dissolves and reconstitutes.

Working with patients, I found different ways to define hospitalization as liminal. Moon Powder, for instance, is a concoction for transformation made of transitional elements. At the moment between waxing and waning when the moon is full in a dark forest penetrated by moonlight, what will be released into the globe at the new moon is captured in a pottery jar. It is a concoction of an ephemeral moment when the tensions of opposites are held in balance so that they can serve to facilitate change. And Moon Powder is only the first example of the magical homeopathic remedies in Dr. Merryandrew's pharmacopeia. The Shield of Light, too, is conceived as magical homeopathy. The body of the patient is enveloped in an isolated enclosure, a place removed from place, which Dr. Merryandrew identifies as a wrinkle in time, a time out of time. In the Shield of Light a patient can find the peace and rest needed to recover strength to go back to the journey on the highway of life. Rupert in his own right, too, is a facilitator of transformations. He, too, works homeopathically. For he serves as an agent of change for the ill with his practice of sweeping first used for chimneys but re-employed to empty patients of pain and poison so that they can be restored to the fullness of life and vitality. And Dr. Merryandrew recognizes in the Harmonies of Healing that music has a magical homeopathic quality that draws the original spark of creation down from the planets and stars into the patient's body and organs to attune or re-attune the patient to a sense of well-being. For as he says, "We are all stardust."

Practicing my magical homeopathy, I have come to recognize and clarify that the experience of liminal reality creates an opening. That opening is at first filled with uncertainty and surrender, which is paradoxically to say that it is filled with a sense of emptiness. Yet in the emptiness there is increased receptivity. And into the emptiness, I have tried with a fanciful magical homeopathy to bring to the experience of being ill some sense of possibility and meaning lightly touched with humor. Instead of regarding illness as meaningless, I have hoped to suggest that in times of illness there can be profound and meaningful significance that affects one's sense of well-being. But I do not burden the message with heaviness or piety; I simply play upon the theme.

When I began to work with Jamie, I did not initially take into account that a puppet has a legacy in the liminal and has by nature a heritage as an agent of transformation. But certainly puppetry has its origin in cultures other than our own where puppets are frequently used in rites of passage. Cultures in which puppets are used in ritual maintain the perspective that everything in the universe is integrally related to everything else and any element in the universe has a dynamic force of its own to influence and change all others. The dynamic principle binding the integral universe is participation. This is the principle behind the sympathetic magic that spawns Dr. Merryandrew's homeopathic remedies. But what has all this got to do with Jamie?

To answer that question in brief, Jamie is the weaver of integral relation par excellence. First of all to enter again into the dispute about whether or not he is real, whether he is an animate or inanimate being, there is a response different than the one he gives. From the perspective of a world view of integral relation, nothing is inanimate. Everything possesses the vitality of being. Nothing is without agency. Children for whom the world is still fresh with vitality know this for they have a natural inclination for participatory consciousness. For children the world is alive and enchanted still. So though they may not admit to it, they implicitly recognize Jamie as an animate being. Though they may protest that he is not real, more often than not they do so paradoxically by arguing with him.

Yet not to overstate the case that participatory consciousness occurs only in children, I need quickly to correct for the possible misunderstanding by clarifying that in our culture children are not alone in their capacity to regard the world with participatory consciousness. Though the sense of a world where everything possesses vitality is more latent in our ordinary awareness, we adults do possess the capacity to see the world with participatory consciousness, as well. When a nurse argues with Jamie and says that she cannot believe that she is arguing with a puppet, she exposes her adult capacity to reinvigorate the world through participatory consciousness.

In fact, in adults the capacity to understand that we live in a universe of integral relation is a measure of the highest order of consciousness, as the great twentieth century scientist attested. Albert Einstein's thought in this regard was written in an exchange of letters he had with Lucien Levy-Bruhl, who was a philosophical anthropologist who developed the notion of the principle of participation as a unique quality in "primitive mentality." Einstein argued that in his conception of relativity the universe is composed of integral relation. Everything influences everything else. Consequently, participatory consciousness is a capacity of the highest order of thinking and not exclusively the quality of "primitive mentality" or the minds of children. So let's face it, Jamie's way of knowing is not just for children.

This may seem, however, to take us adrift from recognizing concretely Jamie's status as an agent of change in the liminal reality of patient experience. Yet in developing the notion of participatory consciousness in relation to Jamie, I am recognizing that just by entering the room, Jamie has the potentiality to affect a change of consciousness. Then he works his own magic on what he finds. He dances into each moment with a patient with total engagement. He finds relations and connections. He plies his own associative logic. With his own cantankerous way of delighting in things, he shapes the time of illness into a rite of passage. Behind his simple imaginations, his purposes are transformation. He touches lightly into the mood of the room with the hope that his small bit of cheer will ripple through the patient's sense of himself and his world of connection. When Jamie sings, "love is something if you give it away" and "it wouldn't be make believe if you believed," he is a diminutive advocate of the grandest of all lessons that love has the power to transform the way we see the world and how we live in community with each other. There is homeopathic magic in that.

With regard to the stories he tells and their pertinence in the context of the liminal reality of hospitalization, Dr. Merryandrew is quite direct about telling patients that all his tales have something to do with transformation. Folktales and fairytales in different cultures are generally recognized as repositories of cultural wisdom about creation, development and change. Yet in his introduction to each tale, Dr. Merryandrew makes clear that the tales he tells are about changes and transformations, as he says:

All my stories are old stories, not because they were told long ago or because they are about things that happened long ago. They are old stories because I learned from the old masters. The old masters knew that life is full of magic and miracle, that sometimes people can turn into animals and sometimes animals can turn into people. They knew that animals and people could communicate with each other, or as we say, they could talk.

The old masters knew that life was full of magic and miracle. They knew... that any path goes down before it goes up and it goes through darkness before it comes to light. They knew we meet many guides and helpers in our lives. Some of these are guides we seek. Some are helpers who show up when we think we are lost, stuck and alone. Sometimes they help us by doing what we ask. Sometimes they guide us by asking us to do something for them.

The old masters knew that life is full of magic and miracle. They knew that there are spirits in the world who watch us even when we do not think that they are there. They knew that kindness and patience are as powerful as judgment and boldness for they invite a spirit to appear to heal a broken body, restore a broken life, and turn our hardships into gifts.

Maybe if we listen to the old stories, we will know what the old masters knew. Maybe if there are more people around who have heard the old stories, there will be more people around who know that life is full of magic and miracle.

If he signals in his introductions that his tales are about transformations that happen in the narrative he has to tell, Dr. Merryandrew also explicitly states at the end of each tale that his tales offer patients opportunities to view their own lives in flux and transition, as he says:

You know, the great thing about these old stories is you can place yourself in them at different stages of your life. That way they give you a sense of where you are in the story of your life. Are you riding across the world to bring back a beautiful princess? Are you trying to recover a hidden chest with something important inside in a far off part of the world? Are you expecting a reward for something you have accomplished? Are you hoping to capture a magical mystical being? Are you in a vat of boiling oil, wondering whether you are going to be turned into a golden being or a bear? Are you about to pick up a golden feather when you have been warned not to? Where are you right now in the story?

You know each time you hear one of the old stories, you can put yourself into it in a different place in the story. One time you may feel it would be thrilling to have the companionship of a wild animal like a wolf. Another time you may feel as if a dear friend has disappeared and you want to go searching for her. Sometimes you may feel you are given an impossible task to complete. Then there are the times in your life that it seems magical agents show up to help you. Every time you hear the story, it becomes new.

You can put yourself somewhere in the story and it tells you something about where you are in your life. Are you deciding whether to choose material possessions or blessings in life? Are you making do with what you have? Are you crying about the hardships you've been through? Is there someone who makes you feel good about yourself even with all your flaws? Do you sometimes feel you are snagged in the roots in the river of life?

So it seems, without setting out to do so, Dr. Merryandrew has developed a practice in which he encourages patients to see their illness and hospitalization as an opportunity, not just as a heavy burden. There is in it the promise of transformation. More than that, there is the opportunity to find meaning and purpose in this liminal time and to deepen one's compassion and empathy for all who suffer. With his tales and folly, Dr. Merryandrew does what he can to facilitate transformation and change, to tease patients toward a sense of meaning and purpose, and to foster compassion and empathy. He does so in his role as Clown/Trickster/Fool whose archetypal purpose is always to increase, inspire and celebrate the vitality of life. Accordingly, I hope at the end, that Dr. Merryandrew and his book have offered you, Reader, a bit of kindling for the fire of your heart.

§ § §

I would like to think that Dr. Farmer, my childhood pediatrician, would appreciate what I do for patients in the hospital. But I am afraid she would not. For after all, she was a no nonsense German doctor. Yet I harbor some hope she would have understood; she might have been more sympathetic than I believe. She did have that wonderfully mysterious Old World room in her house on the other side of the hall from her medical office. In a room with a grand piano and walls lined with books, where even the door becomes a bookcase when closed, one could almost hear someone singing the beautiful lieder of Schubert and Mahler that transport the soul and a gently accented voice whispering the stories of Scheherazade. In such a room, one could dream into the world full of magic and miracle.

If, however, Dr. Farmer would not have lent her support, I hope at least that the little girl in Renoir's painting of a child in a garden, whom I thought for all my childhood was a portrait of Dr. Farmer as a child, I hope at least that she would enjoy what I do.

For the most part, I cannot know if the impact of what I do lasts beyond a moment. It is certainly enough to feel that I have changed a moment for a patient in the hospital. I do not need to know if anything I do has had a lasting effect. For I have seen enough of life to know that sometimes one moment with a stranger one will never see again can resonate for years, even over the course of a whole life. Sometimes I revisit in my own life such moments as touchstones of meaningful encounter. So I wonder now and then if I have had some lasting impact. A few times, I have learned I have.

One morning in the Pediatric unit, a mother who was there with her child came up to me as I entered the unit. Although I did not recognize her, she greeted me warmly. She said she was there that day with her younger son. But she wanted me to know that her older son was in the unit two years earlier and I had come in to be with him. She said he still talked about my visit.

Another day I wrote in my notes for the day:

> The team was just coming out of K___'s room and I had to wait for them to walk past me in the hall. As they did, one of the medical students hung back to talk to me. He said that six years ago he had been a patient in this unit and I came to

see him. He wanted to thank me for that visit. I looked him up in my notes, which I keep religiously each day, and found him there and what I had done for him six years earlier when he was sixteen. It was a thrill to me to hear that I achieved some small lasting impression in the memory of such a fine young man who was on his way to becoming a doctor.

It is true, we never know what even a single encounter may mean in a life. For life is full of magic and miracle.

As reassuring as it is for me as a performer to be recognized and appreciated for what I do, the depth of my commitment to the work has nothing to do with the actors desire for adulation. What motivates me to return each day is the overwhelming intensity of the experience I have in engagement with patients. Frequently I am awed by the feeling of the intimate presence of grace in the vitality of the life of another. I feel there before me is another soul richly endowed with the spark of creation and for a few moments, I am privileged to experience that radiance of being, and to honor and to serve the life. That feeling does not register for me as fulfillment. No, rather I would say I exit with a feeling of wonder and reverence for the preciousness of life.

Sometimes after a full day such as this, as I walk down the hill from the hospital building to the parking lot, I am in a reverie of wonder and reverence. How privileged I am to encounter so many wondrous souls through my work.

Today on the walk out of the hospital, I feel the heat of summer in North Carolina on my back and am blinded by the bright sunlight. The summer heat will be with us for awhile. A starling sings in the ginkgo beside me. I say hello. I see a bluebird on the wire overhead and a cardinal flies by. Chickadees, and sparrows peck in the plantings along the sidewalk. Dragonflies zip through the cars mating and separating. High above a red-tailed hawk screams on an upward draft. A turkey vulture, known to the Cherokee as Peace Eagle, dips its wings and soars in wide circles. Nurses have told me that they have seen foxes out here near their cars when they leave late.

We are high enough on a hill that if it were not for the artificial light at night, this would be a good place to view the stars and yes, listen for the music of the spheres. From this high up I have watched storm fronts roll into the area. By day from the sixth floor of Pediatrics, one can look across the rooftops and get a wide view of the city and feel part of the vastness of the land and sky.

This is where it all begins and ends for me, in the pulse and jubilance that is the celebration of life and creation. I walk out with gratitude to be alive and aware in all this abundance.

Acknowledgements

While responsibility for all deliberate and inadvertent folly in the manuscript is mine alone, the book entire is intended as a paean to those who have inspired me every day in the hospital. They are too many and protected by the laws of patient and professional privacy to be mentioned here by name, but I hope that those among them who see this work will receive it with my deep gratitude. There are some few, however, I do wish to name with regard to the making of the book. First I offer special thanks to my wife, Peggy, and my daughter, Casey, who listened with attention and appreciation to an early reading of the manuscript. A first reading in its own right is a rite of passage for the writer and the book. They lovingly sponsored me through it. To my friend, David Brown, who is a master at manipulating light in the studio and capturing the light in vast landscapes and the sky with his photography, I am most grateful for making the photograph that graces the cover of this book. I hope someday soon the world will see his own book of photographs of landscapes and sky in the West. I am also grateful to my son-in-law, Rory Bradley, for formatting and designing the text. That he did this while working full-time and taking a full load of graduate courses to re-career and parenting fully with Liz to raise their daughter, Josie, seems miraculous to me. Those with whom I corresponded for permission to use the segments of songs in the text, in all instances, were most kind and generous in granting permission. I gratefully acknowledge their permission to reprint the following:

Wrinkle in Time with liner notes from *Beaucatcher Farewell*
Words and Music by Bob Zentz
Copyright © 1979
All Rights Reserved Used by Permission
Reprinted by Permission of Bob Zentz

Magic Penny
Words and Music by Malvina Reynolds
Copyright © 1955, 1959 UNIVERSAL MUSIC CORP.
Copyright Renewed
All Rights Reserved Used by Permission
Reprinted by Permission of Hal Leonard LLC

Slan Abhaile
Words and Music by Tommy Sands
Copyright © 2001
All Rights Reserved Used by Permission
Reprinted by Permission of Tommy Sands

It's Only A Paper Moon
Lyrics by Billy Rose and E.Y. "Yip" Harburg
Music by Harold Arlen
Copyright © 1933 (Renewed) CHAPPELL & CO., INC., GLOCCA MORRA MUSIC and S.A. MUSIC CO.
All Rights for GLOCCA MORRA MUSIC Administered by SHAPIRO, BERNSTEIN & CO., INC
All Rights Reserved
Reprinted by Permission of Hal Leonard LLC

Music of Healing
Words and Music by Tommy Sands
Copyright © 1995
All Rights Reserved Used by Permission
Reprinted by Permission of Tommy Sands

Notes

1. Nortin M. Hadler, *By the Bedside of the Patient: Lessons for the Twenty-First-Century Physician* (Chapel Hill: The University of North Carolina Press, 2016) 10.

2. Victor Turner, *The Ritual Process* (Hammondsworth, Middlesex, England: Penguin Books Ltd., 1969) 81.

3. "Wrinkle in Time" by Bob Zentz.

4. Liner notes from *Beaucatcher Farewell* by Bob Zentz.

5. Liner notes from *Beaucatcher Farewell* by Bob Zentz.

6. "Magic Penny" by Malvina Reynolds.

7. "Slan Abhaile" by Tommy Sands.

8. Thomas Berry, *The Dream of the Earth* (San Francisco, Sierra Club Books, 1988) 131.

9. Maria Popova, "Einstein on Fairy Tales and Education," The Marginalian 03/14/2014, https//www.themarginalian.org/2014/03/14/Einstein-fairy-tales.

10. "It's Only A Paper Moon." Lyrics by Billy Rose and E.Y. "Yip" Harburg. Music by Harold Arlen.

11. "Music of Healing" by Tommy Sands.

12. Mario Livio, *The Golden Ratio: The Story of Phi, the World's Most Astonishing Number* (New York: Broadway Books,

2002) 29.

13. Frederick Buechner, *Telling the Truth: The Gospel as Tragedy, Comedy and Fairy Tale* (San Francisco: Harper and Row, 1977) 57.

14. Rachel Naomi Remen, MD, *My Grandfather's Blessings: Stories of Strength, Refuge, and Belonging* (New York: Riverhead Books, 2000) 2-3.

15. Ibid. 4-5.

16. Ibid. 9.

17. Victoria Sweet, *Slow Medicine: The Way of Healing* (New York: Riverhead Books, 2017) 285.

18. *Children of Paradise: A Film by Marcel Carne*, English trans. Dinah Brooke © 1968 by Lorimer Publishing Limited (New York: Simon and Schuster, 1968) 69.

19. Ibid. 173.